ANATOMY &
STRETCHING FOR
PREGNANCY
& POSTPARTUM

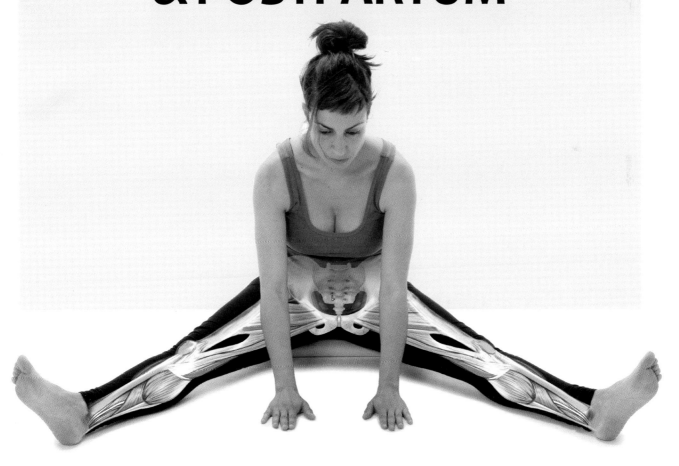

Meyer & Meyer Sport

British Library of Cataloguing in Publication Data
A catalogue record for this book is available from the British Library

Anatomy & Stretching for Pregnancy & Postpartum
Maidenhead: Meyer & Meyer Sport (UK) Ltd., 2023
ISBN: 978-1-78255-255-0

Aachen, Auckland, Beirut, Cairo, Cape Town, Dubai, Hägendorf, Hong Kong, Indianapolis, Maidenhead, Manila, New Delhi, Singapore, Sydney, Tehran, Vienna

Member of the World Sport Publishers' Association (WSPA), www.w-s-p-a.org
Printed in Spain

ISBN: 978-1-78255-255-0
Email: info@m-m-sports.com
www.thesportspublisher.com

Original Spanish edition, *Anatomía & estiramientos para el embarazo y el posparto*, © 2022 Editorial Paidotribo
ISBN: 978-84-9910-749-3
www.paidotribo.com
Email: paidotribo@paidotribo.com

Credits
Cover and interior layout: Annika Naas
Managing editor: Elizabeth Evans
Copy editor: Sarah Tomblin, www.sarahtomblinediting.com
Translation: AAA Translation, www.aaatranslation.com

Project and production: Editorial Paidotribo
Spanish edition: Ángeles Tomé
Text: Mireia Patiño Coll
Scientific review: Mª Dolores Lara Campos, David Martínez Cejudo
Illustrations: Myriam Ferrón
Photos: Nos i Soto
Layout for Spanish edition: Toni Inglès
Models: Ele Rodríguez, Cristina Salvia, Pilar Crespo, Laura Mosquera
Pre-press: Joan Moreno

Introduction

Pregnancy, childbirth, and the postpartum period is a time when great changes occur, both physically and emotionally, in a very short period of time, and to which it is necessary to continuously and progressively adapt.

Gentle physical exercise, combined with stretching, conscious breathing, and relaxation, can help reduce and even make any pain disappear, as well as correct posture, improve your breathing and mood, and help during labor. It is also important to follow a program of gentle exercises and stretches during the postpartum period to recover and strengthen those areas of the body that remain flaccid and looser.

This book is a guide to stretching exercises during both pregnancy and postpartum. The stretches explained in this book should be used to help increase your well-being during this phase and are not meant to improve physical performance. Practicing any form of exercise during pregnancy must be gentle and respectful of the needs and condition of our bodies.

The sections in this book provide general and practical information on anatomy, pregnancy, exercises, breathing and relaxation.

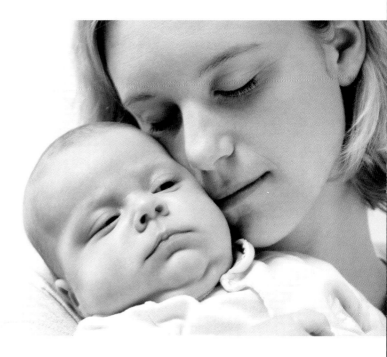

The first section presents a brief introduction to the onset of life and the first symptoms that appear during the first weeks of pregnancy.

Pregnancy and motherhood are unique and wonderful experiences in a woman's life

The second section talks about anatomy and physiology. Physical and emotional changes that arise in each of the three trimesters are explained. This section also presents a monthly guide on fetal development that describes how the baby grows in the mother's womb.

The following five sections cover how to practice stretching. They explain stretching and practice basics during pregnancy, as well as the correct body postures when standing and seated.

The third section, "Stretching During Pregnancy," explains group stretching per pregnancy trimester. The technique, benefits, and precautions are presented for each trimester. It also shows easier or harder variations along with the main image and illustration of the muscles involved in the stretching.

The eighth section talks about postpartum recovery. This section explains the hypopressive exercises for abdominals, pelvic floor activation, transverse abdominal work, and core work. The exercises presented are safe for the abdomen and pelvic floor. Although the exercises are thoroughly detailed, this does not in any way replace the presence of a physical therapist with experience of the pelvic floor.

Finally, respiratory and relaxation techniques that are helpful for developing our own resources to experience pregnancy, childbirth, and the postpartum period in a happy and lively manner are explained.

Mireia Patiño Coll
IYTA (International Yoga Teachers Association)
Yoga Instructor
Stretching Technician

Contents

4

How to Use This Book

Pregnancy/Postpartum stage

Exercise name

Technique description

Anatomical illustration

See video of the exercise

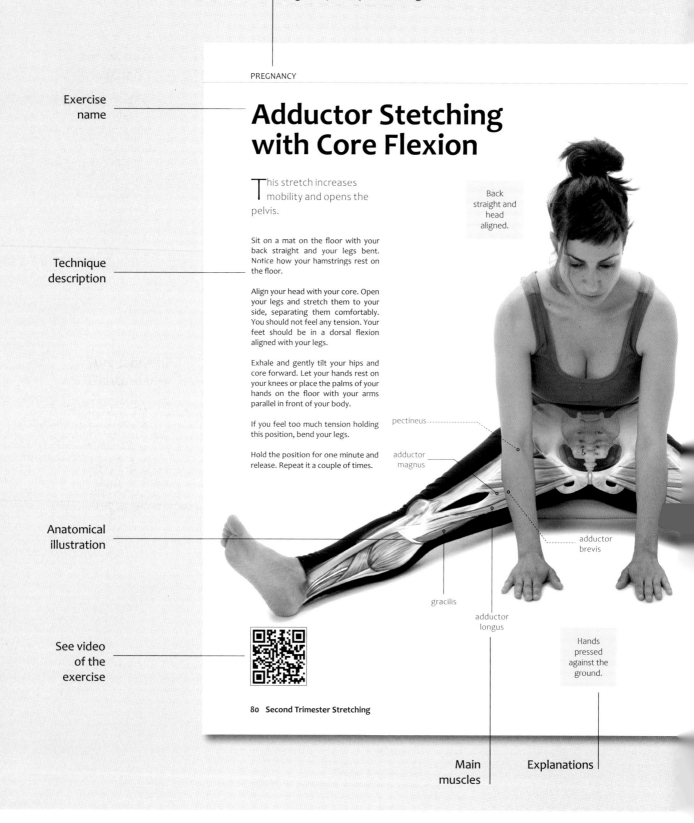

PREGNANCY

Adductor Stetching with Core Flexion

This stretch increases mobility and opens the pelvis.

Sit on a mat on the floor with your back straight and your legs bent. Notice how your hamstrings rest on the floor.

Align your head with your core. Open your legs and stretch them to your side, separating them comfortably. You should not feel any tension. Your feet should be in a dorsal flexion aligned with your legs.

Exhale and gently tilt your hips and core forward. Let your hands rest on your knees or place the palms of your hands on the floor with your arms parallel in front of your body.

If you feel too much tension holding this position, bend your legs.

Hold the position for one minute and release. Repeat it a couple of times.

Back straight and head aligned.

pectineus

adductor magnus

adductor brevis

gracilis

adductor longus

Hands pressed against the ground.

80 Second Trimester Stretching

Main muscles

Explanations

6

Associated
benefits

Main exercise
variations

Practice
period

Green: Practice during this trimester
Green: Practice highly recommended during this trimester
Red: Do not practice during this trimester

How to access additional content

In addition to the content published on the pages of this book, *Anatomy & Stretching for Pregnancy and Postpartum*, includes additional content with 36 video tutorials. It is the most complete work on the subject matter. In order to access this content, scan the QR code on each page with your mobile phone.

Variants

Stretching of posterior muscles of the body with legs bent

This variant can be practiced when you feel tension in the posterior part of the back or lack of flexibility in your hamstring muscles.

Sit on the floor with your legs bent and resting the heels of your feet on the floor. Your back should be straight and your core resting on your sit bones. Place your hands on the corresponding foot.

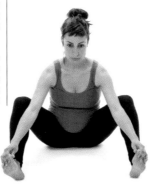

* Stretches and strengthens the muscles of the back and legs.
* Increases mobility in the pelvis.

⚠

* If there is tension in the lumbar part of the back or lack of flexibility in the legs, you must sit on a block or a folded blanket and extend your legs until you do not feel tension.
* If you have spinal injuries, practice with your legs bent.
* Avoid excessive stretching so that the pubic symphysis does not stretch excessively.

Includes videos and tutorials

Accessible on all pages where the QR code appears

Internet connection is necessary to access the multimedia content.

Adductor stretching with support

Deepen the stretch with the help of a chair. Sit on the floor facing the front of the chair. Extend your legs while keeping your elbows on the seat. You can also use your hands to hold the back of the chair.

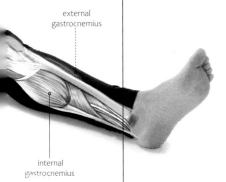

external gastrocnemius

internal gastrocnemius

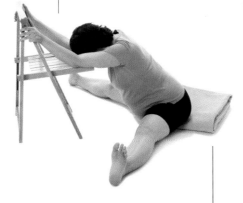

Adductor Stretching with Core Flexion   81

Precautions and contraindications

Exercise adaptations

Introduction to Pregnancy

Big and profound changes can occur during pregnancy that can cause uncertainties and concerns. Having knowledge about what we can expect during this period will help us better and more positively address the needs in each stage.

In this introductory chapter, we focus on the beginning of life and explain the first symptoms at the beginning of pregnancy. Changes that occur on a physical and emotional level are also briefly explained.

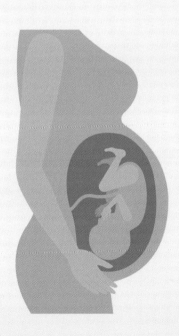

The Beginning of Life

The fascinating adventure of life, which begins on a microscopic level, originates when an egg and a sperm cell join together to form a single cell. The zygote, which occurs in fertilization, will contain half the genetic information from the father and the other half from the mother. For conception to happen, three favorable events are required: ovulation, fertilization, and implantation of the fertilized egg in the uterine wall.

The Menstrual Cycle and Ovulation

The time between the first day of your period and the first day of your following period is called a menstrual cycle. Normally, a menstrual cycle usually lasts about 28 days, although frequency varies from woman to woman. Periods of 21 to 35 days are considered normal. Ovulation occurs during the middle of the menstrual cycle when the egg leaves the ovary and is when a woman is fertile.

At the beginning of each menstrual cycle, about 100 or 150 eggs begin to mature inside the ovary in sacs called follicles. By mid-month, the pituitary gland produces a luteinizing hormone (lutropin or LH) that, along with the follicle-stimulating hormone (FSH), stimulates follicle rupture and egg release (ovulation). In addition, increased lutropin will induce secretion of the hormone progesterone. This hormone prepares the mucosa of the wall of the uterus (endometrium) to accommodate a possible zygote or blastocyst.

The egg, which has left the ovary, begins a small journey along the fallopian tube. Within a period of about 12 hours, the egg can be fertilized. If conception does not occur, the egg dies, and the lining of the uterine wall is expelled; this is when menstruation occurs.

Some signs that you are ovulating.

Menstrual Cycle

If your menstrual cycle is regular, ovulation will occur during the middle of the cycle.

"Average Pain"

Twenty-five percent of women notice pain in the lower abdomen in their ovaries when ovulation occurs.

Mucus

Mucus from the cervix becomes more transparent, thin, and moist.

Body Temperature

The increase in progesterone causes a slight increase in body temperature: from about 97.5 to 98 °F (appx. 36 to 37 °C).

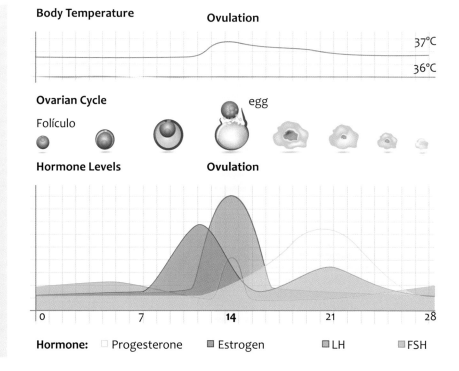

Menstrual Cycle

Body Temperature — Ovulation — 37°C — 36°C

Ovarian Cycle — Folículo — egg

Hormone Levels — Ovulation

0   7   14   21   28

Hormone: ☐ Progesterone   ■ Estrogen   ■ LH   ■ FSH

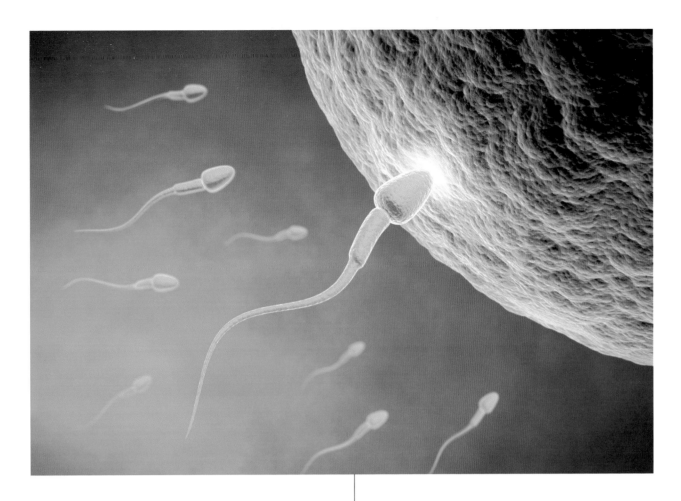

A sperm is 0.05 millimeters long. When they reach the wall of the egg, they must go through two layers. The first one that reaches the nucleus will be the one that merges with the egg.

The sperm race and fertilization

Fertilization is the union of an egg with a sperm. For it to occur, millions of sperm released in ejaculation need to begin a long race through the vagina, the uterus, and the fallopian tubes to finally reach the egg.

Only about 200 sperm will reach the fallopian tubes. The distance they have to travel to reach the egg is about six to seven inches, which, considering their microscopic size, is quite an accomplishment. The quickest ones take about 45 minutes to arrive, and the slowest ones take about 12 hours. Fertilization can occur even if it is two to three days before ovulation, which is possible since sperm can survive up to four days inside the uterus.

When the sperm reach the wall of the egg, they have to go through two layers: the outer layer (radiant crown) and the zona pellucida. The first one that reaches the nucleus emits a substance that acts as a barrier so that the other sperm cannot enter. The winning sperm merges with the egg, loses its tail, and its head begins to grow. This is when fertilization occurs.

The egg and the sperm will each provide 23 chromosomes and will form a new cell with 46 chromosomes called a zygote. A few hours later, the zygote begins to split and form new cells: the blastomeres. About four days after fertilization, a solid ball formed by about 32 blastomeres can be seen. From that moment on, the initial cell will be called a morula.

Pregnancy

Two weeks after menstruation, egg fertilization from a sperm can occur. The fertilized egg will begin a journey through the fallopian tube to the uterus where it will adhere. Once the blastocyst is established in the uterus, pregnancy and embryo development begins, which will last an average of 266 days from the moment conception occurs.

Blastocyst Journey and Its Establishment in the Uterus

The fertilized egg, which has continued its journey down the fallopian tube, reaches the uterus. During this time, the morula grows and becomes a sphere called a blastocyst consisting of three parts: an internal cell mass that will form the fetus, cells that will form the future placenta (trophoblast), and an internal fluid-filled cavity (blastocoel).

On the other hand, progesterone production, which reaches its highest level between days five and seven after ovulation, favors blood vessel development of the endometrium and its glands. The latter become bulkier and full of nutrients (glycogen).

This coincides with the arrival of the blastocyst, which will float freely for a few days through the uterus until it adheres to the endometrium. The embryo, attached to the wall of the uterus, begins to develop and remove the nutrients and oxygen provided by the endometrium.

Importantly, implantation is not always completed. It is estimated that 40 percent of blastocysts never get to attach to the uterus, so they die and are removed in the following menstruation.

Once the blastocyst is implanted, the placenta begins to develop, which is the organ that will provide oxygen and nutrients to the growing baby as well as eliminate waste substances.

Pregnancy begins when the blastocyst is implanted and lasts until the day of birth: a total of 266 days from egg fertilization. If calculated from the first day of your last period, add 14 days, which equals 280 days. Use the following formula to determine the PDD (Probable Date of Delivery):

PDD = Last period + 9 months + 7 days

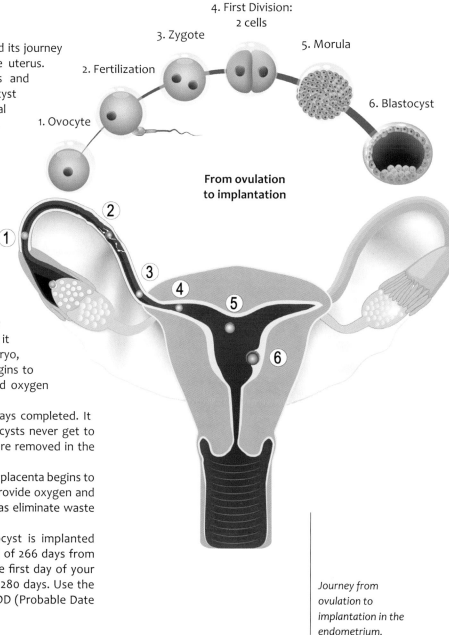

1. Ovocyte
2. Fertilization
3. Zygote
4. First Division: 2 cells
5. Morula
6. Blastocyst

From ovulation to implantation

Journey from ovulation to implantation in the endometrium.

First Symptoms of Pregnancy

One of the first symptoms that many women perceive is the "feeling of being pregnant." This is due to the major hormonal changes that occur. In addition to the absence of menstruation, there are a number of revealing signs of pregnancy, such as nausea, tiredness, breast tenderness, frequent urination, and changes in taste and smell.

Absence of Menstruation

If a woman's cycle is usually regular, missing your period is a classic symptom of pregnancy. Lack of menstrual bleeding is called amenorrhea and is usually the most obvious sign. However, there may be other reasons for delayed menstruation, for instance, stress, anxiety, shock, illness, travel, or even weight loss.

Fatigue

The onset of fatigue and drowsiness at any time of the day is a frequent symptom. Many women experience an irresistible urge to nap after eating or the need to go to bed early at night. This is probably to do with progesterone, as the level in the blood increases, creating a calming and sedative effect on the body.

Morning Sickness

Nausea accompanied by vomiting is usually one of the most bothersome symptoms early in pregnancy. It usually appears during the fifth week, but there are women who suffer from this during their second week. These symptoms tend to decrease and usually disappear between weeks 15 and 16 of pregnancy.

One possible cause is an increase in hormone levels circulating in the blood. One of the causes of nausea is thought to be the placental release of the human chorionic gonadotropin hormone (hCG) known as the "pregnancy hormone." This hormone is the one detected in pregnancy tests.

Breast Sensitivity

Breast augmentation and sensitivity is one of the earliest signs. You may feel heaviness, itching, sore nipples, and even a tingling sensation, all of which will disappear within a few weeks.

From the moment the blastocyst is implanted, hCG is produced in the uterus. This hormone is the one that can be detected in pregnancy tests.

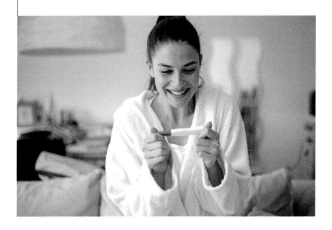

Frequent Urge to Urinate

Many women feel a frequent desire to urinate, which occurs because of the distension of the uterus pressing against the bladder. This can be felt from the first week after conception.

Change in Taste and Smell

A change in taste and smell is a common feeling for some women. It is common that smells or tastes you liked before can now be unpleasant. You may feel an exaggerated increase in smell sensitivity and consequent rejection to certain foods. Some women also have a metallic taste in their mouth when eating.

Pregnancy test kit.

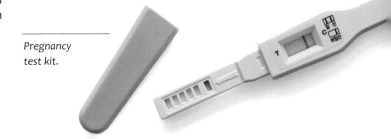

A Time of Change

During pregnancy, many changes are experienced at both a physical and emotional level. Part of this process of change is due to the large increase in hormonal secretion that occurs in the body during these months. To deal with discomfort with a positive attitude, it is helpful to know what the changes are and their causes.

Physical Changes

From the moment of conception, the body begins to adapt to supply nutrients and oxygen to a future life. Physical changes occur internally due to increased hormone production as well as external changes, which are more noticeable, such as larger breasts and belly.

Internally, there are three important changes that happen to the circulatory system, respiratory process, and metabolism.

The changes in the circulatory system are vast. Blood volume increases significantly. By weeks 34 to 36 of pregnancy it will have increased by 40 to 50 percent. The heartbeat accelerates by 20 to 40 percent and blood pressure is altered, which tends to drop to its lowest level in the middle of pregnancy.

As for the respiratory process, pregnant women will need a higher level of oxygen. In the last trimester of pregnancy, the enlarged uterus pushes the diaphragm upwards, which rises about an inch and a half. This is compensated by a widening of the ribs due to relaxation of the intercostal ligaments. As your pregnancy progresses, constant chest breathing will become increasingly important.

Metabolism also changes. Blood sugar levels in the mother's blood may fall because the baby needs glucose and nutrients, which it draws from the bloodstream. When glucose levels drop, the mother may feel hungry and even anxious to eat.

On the outside, the most important change is the increased size of the belly and breasts, although there may be noticeable variations in the nails, hair, and skin.

You will notice that the breasts will become fuller and tender from the beginning of pregnancy. Nipples darken and become more prominent. As pregnancy progresses, the veins in the breasts become more visible and larger.

Your nails and hair may grow faster, your hair may grow stronger and greasier, and skin may look softer and brighter. Other skin changes may include the linea nigra, acne, and itching of the hands and feet. It is normal for many of these alterations to disappear after birth.

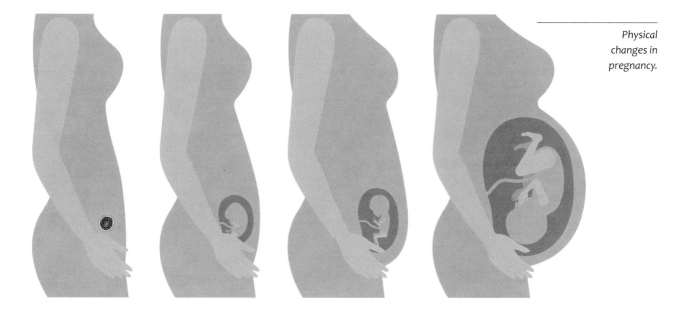

Physical changes in pregnancy.

PREGNANCY HORMONES

HORMONE	ACTION	EFFECTS
Human Chorionic Gonadotropin (hCG)	Causes the ovary to produce more progesterone. Prevents menstruation.	It is thought to be responsible for morning sickness.
Progesterone	Relaxes smooth muscles and sustains pregnancy.	Reinforces and prepares the pelvic wall for labor. Relaxes certain ligaments and muscles in the body. Prepares breasts for breastfeeding.
Estrogen	Helps prepare the uterus lining for pregnancy.	Maintains the health of the genital tract, breasts, and reproductive organs.
Calcitonin	Increases vitamin D synthesis and preserves calcium.	Maintains stable bone and calcium levels.
Relaxin	Relaxes pelvic joints.	It relaxes the cervix, the pelvic muscles, Ligaments, and joints.
Oxytocin	Starts uterus contractions.	Facilitates birth and breastfeeding.

Emotional Changes

In less than nine months, the life of the future mom will change entirely so, during this time, it is normal to go through moments of happiness and euphoria but also to feel doubt, fear, and concern.

Feelings will change depending on your mood. It is therefore important to practice a gentle sport, to stretch, to be part of a group for childbirth preparation, learn to breathe well, take walks in nature, etc. All this will help you maintain a positive attitude. It will predispose you to a better mood and help you feel more confident during childbirth.

Finally, during the postpartum period, physical changes will start to disappear. During this new stage, the mother may feel overwhelmed as, on an emotional level, she will have to face concerns and insecurities about the upbringing of her newborn, in addition to recovering muscle tone. Rest, healthy eating, and exercise will greatly contribute the return to normal and enjoyment of the newborn's arrival.

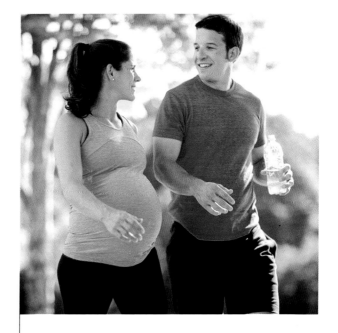

Walking and exercise during pregnancy maintains a positive attitude and improves your mood.

I'm Going to Be a Mom

Knowing you're about to be a mother can be one of the most intense emotions experienced in life. In a few months, the future mother's life will change considerably as the arrival of a baby is an immense responsibility.

Being a Mom: Responsibility and Love

The experience of being a mom begins nine months before delivery. When receiving the news of the pregnancy, you will begin to experience feelings of love toward the life that is growing, although it will not be until a time after birth when the bonds with the baby and maternal love appear definitively and safely. A child's arrival is forever, no matter what. In the future, the mother's life will change completely. Everything that is superfluous will begin to feel less important as dedicating your time to your children takes up an most of your everyday life.

As your baby grows, being a mom goes beyond feeding, dressing, and loving them. The mother as well as the father will become role models.

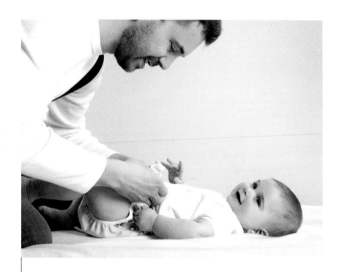

Caring for your baby creates a very positive bond.

Being a mom brings a lot of happiness and good times.

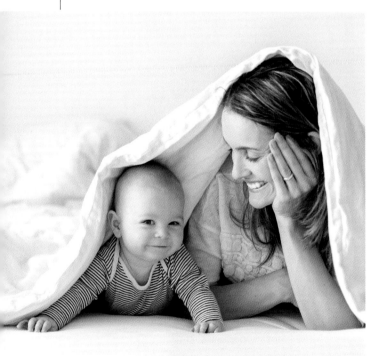

The Couple's Role

Sharing your pregnancy with your partner right from the start creates an opportunity for them to feel included in this wonderful experience. In addition, by actively participating in the whole process, you will allow them to create links with the future baby from the very beginning.

If the decision has been to carry out the pregnancy alone or if the future mother does not have someone to support her during all these months, one option would be to have the help of a birth assistant or a private midwife. A birth assistant is the person who provides emotional assistance to women throughout the pregnancy, birth, and postpartum period.

Pregnancy, childbirth, and postpartum are months of intense change and activity when women need to feel supported and understood. The couple's role, or in their absence, the role of a midwife, relative, or friend, can be a great help in making the woman feel better emotionally.

Giving Birth

Childbirth is intense labor, but it can be experienced in a pleasant manner. This depends on the adequate segregation of three essential hormones: oxytocin, endorphins, and adrenaline.

Oxytocin, also known as the love hormone, is produced in the hypothalamus in small doses throughout pregnancy and increases as labor approaches. This hormone, along with prolactin, are responsible for the uterine contractions during childbirth. It also regulates maternal behavior, attachment, and empathy.

Endorphins are biological opiate substances that relieve pain and promote relaxation. It is important for the future mother to give birth in a relaxed and intimate place in order to segregate this substance.

Finally, adrenaline is the hormone necessary for labor. Its highest level is reached during the last contractions before the baby is born. It allows you to be alert and have maximum energy during labor.

For childbirth to be a natural and positive experience, it is important to know what to expect during this wonderful moment. Also, choosing a childbirth method will allow you to have the necessary physical and psychological resources when the time comes to give birth.

Tips for Mom-To-Be

Motherhood is a change in lifestyle. The arrival of a baby requires a high capacity of adaptation and a lot of devotion to the bay during their first years of life. The baby will need to be cared for with a lot of affection and encouragement to establish safe bonds, which are vital for proper brain development.

New challenges will have to be faced in the way you live, so this is a great time to take care of yourself. A good start, even before you decide to have a child, is to start changing unhealthy habits with ones that strengthen your health and energy including:

Diet. It must be varied and balanced. We need to reduce processed foods and incorporate more fruit, vegetables, and foods with fiber into our diet.

Tobacco, alcohol, and drugs. It is a good time to quit smoking as tobacco can affect the unborn child. Alcohol and drugs pose a risk in the first few weeks of pregnancy.

Physical exercise. Practicing a sport is the best way to prevent disease. It provides numerous benefits both on a physical level (healthy weight, greater flexibility, and endurance) as well as on a mental level (greater self-esteem, improved mood, and the feeling of well-being).

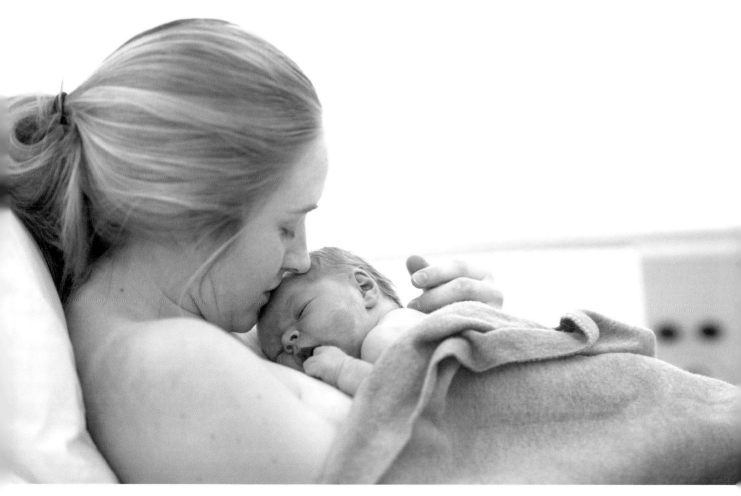

Anatomy and Physiology

Basic knowledge of the anatomy that makes up the skeletal and muscular system is necessary to understand the movements and stretches to be practiced. Understanding how the respiratory system works helps you breathe more consciously.

This chapter presents the basic anatomy and physiology necessary to understand the physical changes along with the mental and emotional changes that occur during pregnancy and postpartum. All of these will be explained by trimester in this section.

The Skeletal System

The skeletal system is a set of bony parts that gives structure to the human to support and protect the organs of the body. It is responsible for movement, along with the muscular system. Within the skeletal system, we find two fundamental bone structures: the spine and the pelvic girdle. These two structures change during pregnancy and childbirth, so it is very important to understand them.

The Spine

It is a longitudinal bony structure that runs from the skull to the pelvis. Its mission is to protect the spinal cord, support the body's position, and help maintain the center of gravity.

It consists of 33 vertebrae, of which, during adulthood, nine fuse forming the sacrum and coccyx, leaving 26 vertebrae. The spine can be divided into five regions according to the vertebrae structure: cervical with 7 vertebrae, thoracic with 12 vertebrae, lumbar with 5 vertebrae, sacral with 5 fused together, and coccyx with 4 fused together.

Between the vertebrae are the intervertebral discs. These are pads of fibrocartilage that, besides being resistant to compression, provide flexibility and shock absorption.

There are four natural curves in the spine: cervical, thoracic, lumbar, and sacral. The curvatures of the cervical and lumbar regions with anterior convexity are called lordosis. The curvatures of the dorsal and sacral region with anterior concavity are called kyphosis.

The spine can perform four movements: forward flexion, backward flexion or extension, lateral flexion, and rotation. Depending on the thickness of the disc and the shape of the vertebrae, the range of motion will be greater or lesser.

Spinal changes in pregnant women. As the fetus grows during pregnancy, the belly increases forward. This causes the center of gravity to shift and changes the curvature of the spine. Progressively, lumbar hyperlordosis and dorsal kyphosis are formed in pregnant woman as a compensation for these variations.

Overloading of the vertebral bodies and the muscles of the back can lead to lumbar, pelvic, and sciatic pain. Dorsal pain may also occur due to contractures in the dorsal muscles. This can be avoided by understanding one's own body position and maintaining good posture when standing and sitting.

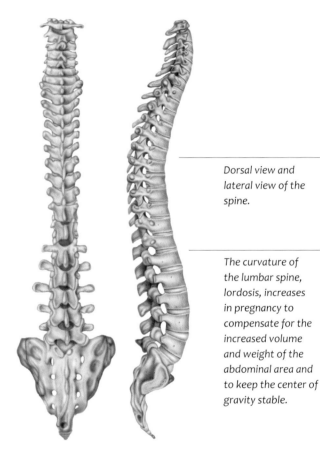

Dorsal view and lateral view of the spine.

The curvature of the lumbar spine, lordosis, increases in pregnancy to compensate for the increased volume and weight of the abdominal area and to keep the center of gravity stable.

The Pelvic Girdle

The pelvic girdle is a bony structure shaped like a large ring. It is made up of four bones: two coxal bones, right and left, the sacrum and the coccyx. Each of the coxal bones consists of a fusion of three bones: the ilium, the hamstring, and the pubis.

The pelvis consists of the pelvic girdle, the cavity it contains, and the lower region of the core where it attaches to the legs. The structure of the female pelvis is different from the male pelvis because of its role in pregnancy and childbirth.

The center of gravity, where the total body weight is concentrated, can be found in the pelvis. In pregnancy, the pelvis naturally rotates forward by generating an anterior pelvic incline and causing a shortening of the flexor hip muscles, the rectus femoris, and the spinal erectors.

In addition, the activity of progesterone and relaxin during pregnancy causes pelvic ligaments to become more laxative, empowering muscle, joint, and ligament mobility. Changing the shape of the pelvis during labor facilitates the baby's passage.

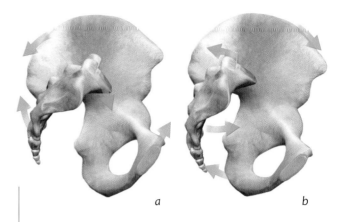

Intrinsic pelvis movements:
a) nutation and b) counternutation.

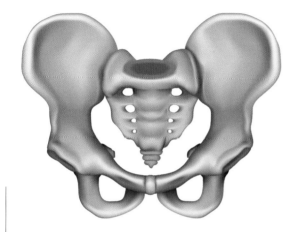

The bone pelvis consists of the left and right coxal bones, the sacrum, and the coccyx.

Pelvic Movements

There are two groups of pelvic movements: intrinsic and extrinsic. Intrinsic movements are those that occur when the pelvis moves only at the expense of its own joints, such as the nutation and counternutation of the sacrum and iliac seen in the sagittal plane (profile).

The sacrum is nutated at the time of childbirth. It is an important movement where the coccyx moves away from the pubis and slightly rises while the top of the sacrum tilts forward. This tilting movement of the sacrum facilitates the passage of the baby's head through the upper strait of the pelvis.

Extrinsic movements are those that occur in relation to the other contiguous structures.

In the sagittal plane, anteversion occurs when the anterior superior iliac spine (ASIS) moves down and forward and the hamstrings move backward, creating greater lumbar curvature. Retroversion is the opposite movement. The ASIS moves back and upward and the hamstrings move forward resulting in a loss of lumbar curvature.

Both external and internal tilts can be performed in the frontal plane. The pelvis is laterally elevated over the hips in these two movements.

The pelvis can perform horizontal twisting movements over the hip (internal and external rotations) in the horizontal plane.

Extrinsic pelvis movements:
a) sagittal plane
b) frontal plane
c) horizontal plane.

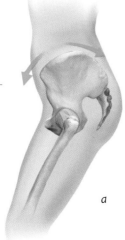
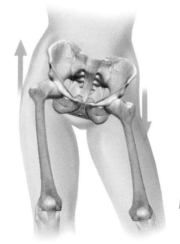
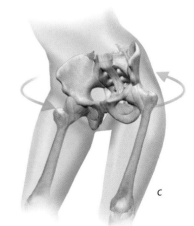

The Muscular System

There are three types of muscles in the body depending on their cell structure and location: the heart muscle, smooth muscles, and skeletal muscles. In this chapter, we will only study the skeletal muscles as they are the ones responsible for movement.

Skeletal Muscles

Skeletal muscles, also called striated muscles or voluntary muscles, are made up of tissue with contractile ability that allows the skeleton to move. We maintain our body posture thanks to these muscles adjusting their position. This way, they can stabilize the joints and keep us upright.

Its living unit is the muscle cell called fiber. These are long, striated cells that are wrapped by a connective tissue (fascia or myofascial tissue) called the endomysium.

In addition to the myofascial tissue, there are two types of fibrous connective tissue found in the muscles: the aponeurosis and the tendons. Aponeuroses are fibrous membranes in the form of a flattened sheet (made up mainly of collagen fibers) which, like the tendon, are used for muscle insertion into the bones. Tendons are connective tissue that insert skeletal muscles into the bones. They allow movement by transmitting the strength of the contraction of the muscle to the bone.

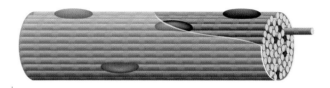

Muscle fibers are made up of myofibrils—which are the contractile element—an external membrane called the sarcolemma, the sarcoplasm or internal fluid, and the internal cellular organs.

Movement

We can move because of the contraction capacity of muscle fibers in the muscles. Muscle fibers contain myofibrils that are formed by a contractile functional unit, the sarcomere. When a muscle is shortened due to lack of exercise or by recurrent poor position, it loses sarcomeres. On the other hand, when we assiduously stretch, the muscle produces more sarcomeres, thus lengthening it.

Muscle contraction is a process by which the muscle becomes tense, and changes its length (isotonic traction) or remains the same length (isometric contraction).

Isotonic contractions are the most common in physical activities, sports, and everyday life. They are further divided into concentric and eccentric contractions. Concentric contractions occur when the muscle shortens and the insertion points of the muscle come closer. An example is when we lift a weight with our biceps. Eccentric contractions occur when the muscle lengthens and slows the movement.

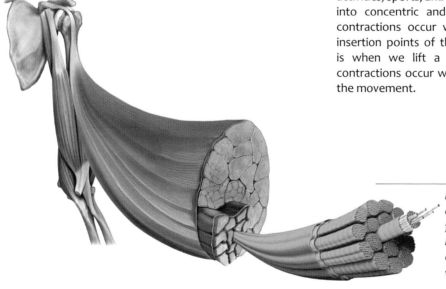

Muscle fibers are wrapped in the endomysium. These are grouped into fascicles wrapped by the perimysium. Many fascicles will form the muscle that is enveloped by the epimysium. This, fused with the tendon, will adhere to the bone.

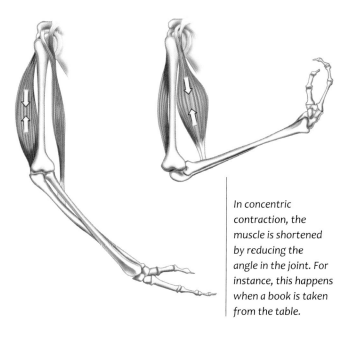

In concentric contraction, the muscle is shortened by reducing the angle in the joint. For instance, this happens when a book is taken from the table.

The Abdominal Wall

The abdominal cavity is located between muscle formations: the upper part formed by the diaphragm (which separates it from the chest cavity), the lower part formed by the pelvic diaphragm and the muscles that form the abdominal walls.

The muscles forming the abdominal walls are classified into three areas: posterior (lumbar square, psoas, and iliopsoas), lateral (transverse and superior and inferior oblique), and anterior (straight and pyramidal). These muscles protect the abdominal viscera and allow us to maintain proper posture by stabilizing the pelvis and lumbar spine. They are also involved in core flexion, rotation, and lateralization movements.

In pregnancy, the expansion of the uterus causes the ab muscles to distend. Normally, the abdominal wall can accommodate the expansion but, in some cases, the rectus abdominis becomes separated excessively, causing a separation called diastasis recti. This may appear physiologically during pregnancy and is usually resolved

gradually during the first eight weeks after delivery. If not, hypopressive and abdominal muscle strengthening exercises can be performed for recovery.

The Pelvic Diaphragm

The pelvic floor, or pelvic diaphragm, is made up of very small layers of muscles and connective tissue that hold the pelvic and abdominal organs together and close the lower abdominal cavity. In addition to being a support for these structures, it helps with urinary and fecal continence.

The pelvic organs can be divided into three compartments: anterior (bladder and urethra), medius (uterus and vagina), and posterior (rectum, anal canal, and sphincter).

During pregnancy, the increased volume in the uterus has a significant effect on the pelvic floor, which is subjected to increased pressure. In addition, hormones released during pregnancy (such as relaxin) cause ligaments in the perineal and abdominal region to become excessively relaxed.

During pregnancy and postpartum, it is necessary to strengthen the pelvic floor through gentle training. Toning these muscles prevents prolapse problems and urinary incontinence.

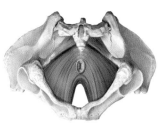

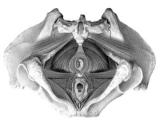

The pelvic floor muscles are located between the pubic bone and the coccyx. They are a structure of muscles and connective tissue that enclose the pelvis at the bottom.

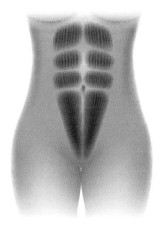

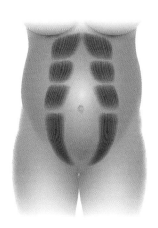

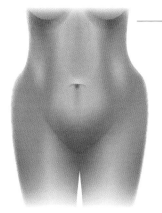

Diastasis recti is the separation of the rectus abdominis muscles as a result from stretching the linea alba. It usually appears physiologically in the third trimester of pregnancy.

The Muscles of the Body

The muscular system allows us to perform the movements of the body. The following are the muscles that are relevant to stretching practice.

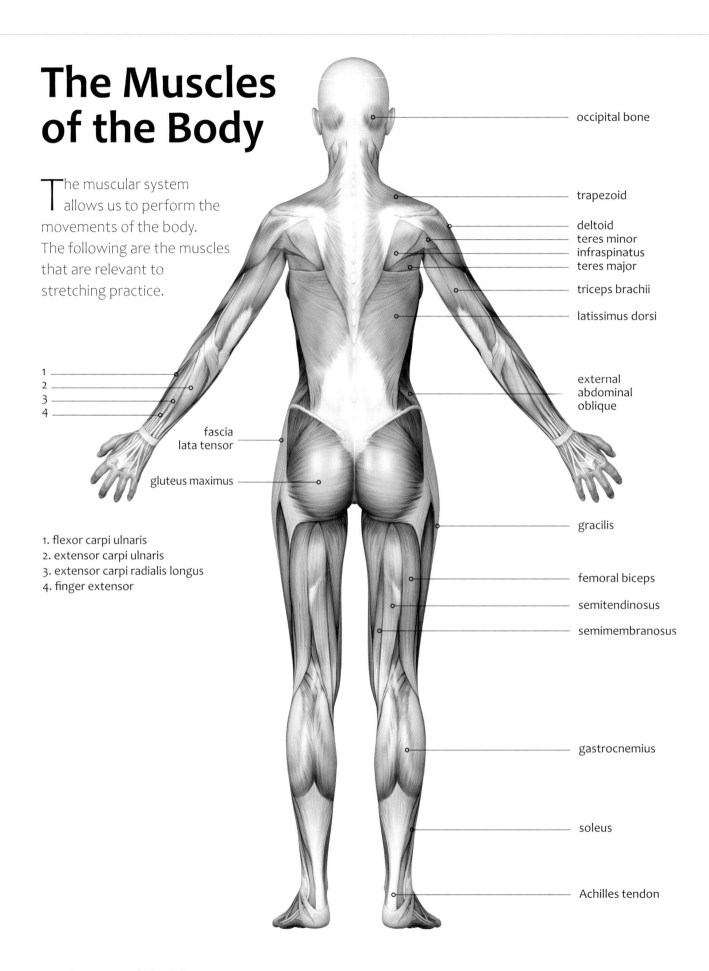

occipital bone

trapezoid

deltoid
teres minor
infraspinatus
teres major

triceps brachii

latissimus dorsi

external abdominal oblique

fascia lata tensor

gluteus maximus

gracilis

femoral biceps

semitendinosus

semimembranosus

gastrocnemius

soleus

Achilles tendon

1
2
3
4

1. flexor carpi ulnaris
2. extensor carpi ulnaris
3. extensor carpi radialis longus
4. finger extensor

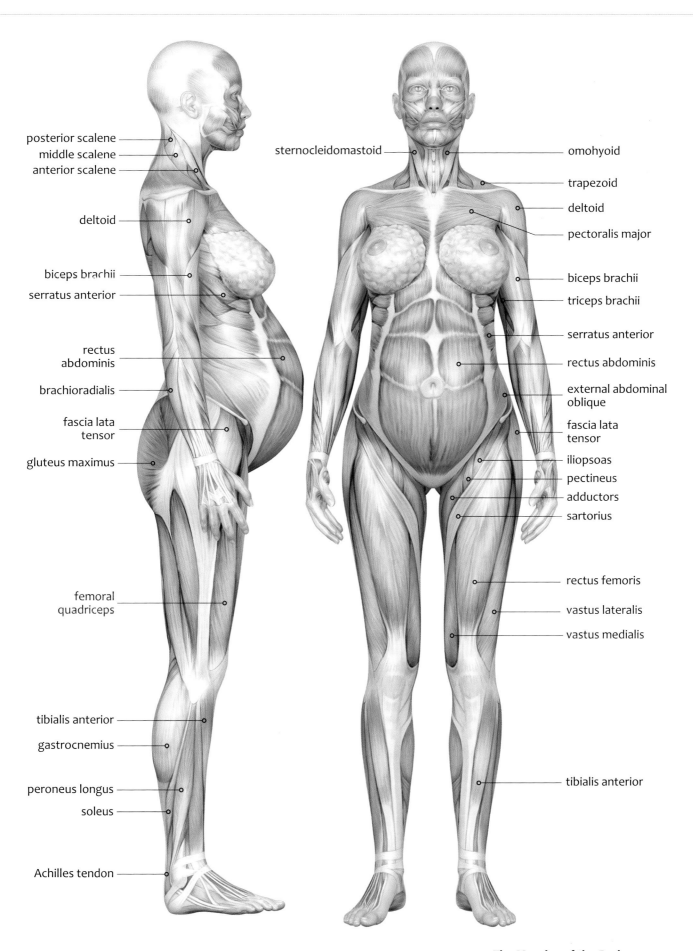

posterior scalene

middle scalene

anterior scalene

sternocleidomastoid

omohyoid

trapezoid

deltoid

deltoid

pectoralis major

biceps brachii

biceps brachii

serratus anterior

triceps brachii

serratus anterior

rectus
abdominis

rectus abdominis

brachioradialis

external abdominal
oblique

fascia lata
tensor

fascia lata
tensor

gluteus maximus

iliopsoas

pectineus

adductors

sartorius

rectus femoris

vastus lateralis

femoral
quadriceps

vastus medialis

tibialis anterior

gastrocnemius

peroneus longus

soleus

tibialis anterior

Achilles tendon

The Muscles of the Body   25

The Respiratory System

The respiratory system, along with the cardiovascular system, provides our body with oxygen and, in turn, expels carbon dioxide. During pregnancy, the respiratory system is altered due to hormonal and anatomical changes.

The Organs of the Respiratory System

The respiratory system consists of hollow organs (the mouth, nose, pharynx, larynx) and channels through which air passes from outside to inside the lungs (the trachea, bronchi, bronchioles).

The structure of the respiratory system can be divided into the airways or breathing channels and the lungs.

The airways are the nasal passages, the pharynx, the larynx, the trachea, and the primary bronchi. The main function of these organs is to transport and facilitate air passage into the lungs. They also serve other functions: the nostrils filter, warm, and humidify the air; the larynx prevents the passage of food and directs air toward the trachea. The bronchi distribute air to both lungs.

The lungs are two organs made up of an elastic tissue, the secondary bronchi, the tertiary bronchi, and the bronchioles. These last three constitute the bronchial tree. The smaller bronchioles make their way into the alveoli, small sacs (0.3 millimeters) where gas exchange with the blood takes place. Oxygen, which is obtained through inhalation, passes into the blood through tiny blood capillaries found in the alveoli. Carbon dioxide goes through these capillaries into the alveoli and is expelled through exhalation.

During gas exchange, the diaphragm is contracted downwards when inhaling.

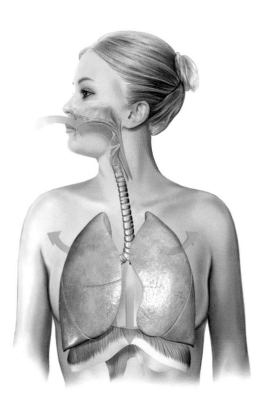

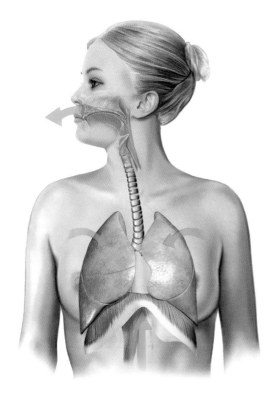

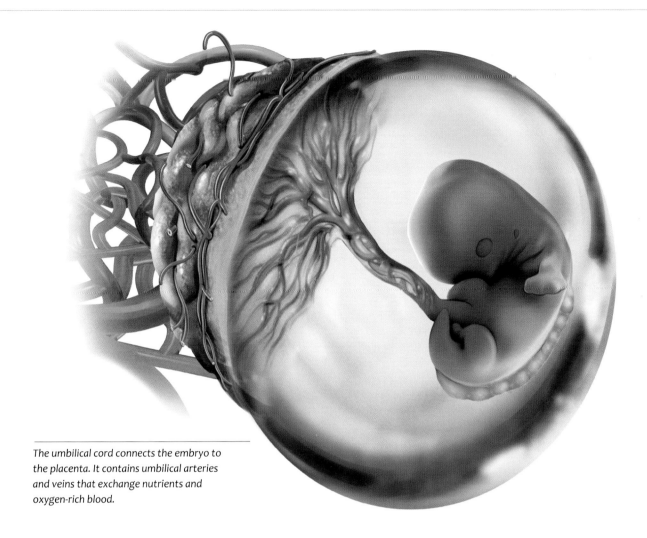

The umbilical cord connects the embryo to the placenta. It contains umbilical arteries and veins that exchange nutrients and oxygen-rich blood.

Respiratory Muscles

The most important respiratory muscles are the diaphragm, the intercostal muscles, and the abdominal muscles.

The diaphragm and intercostal muscles are used in inhalation. Air enters the lungs when the diaphragm contracts and moves downward while the external intercostal muscles lift the ribs and sternum, widening the rib cage. The increased chest volume creates a negative pressure, which causes inhalation to occur and air to enter the lungs.

Exhalation occurs naturally. The muscles involved in inhalation relax and the lung, which is an elastic tissue, recovers its shape when the rib cage is contracted. Abdominal muscles are involved in conscious and forced exhalations.

Pregnancy and Breathing

In pregnancy, as the uterus enlarges, the intestinal organs move toward the diaphragm, which, when pushed upward, rises approximately four centimeters. As a result, the anteroposterior and transverse diameters of the chest increase, stretching the ribs forward, and to the sides. This is why during the last three months of pregnancy, you will notice your breathing located more in the chest cavity and will be shallower and more frequent.

Throughout pregnancy, it is important to be aware of your breathing, starting with your natural breathing and working with diaphragmatic and thoracic breathing, which will allow you to promote better oxygenation of the blood and adequate carbon dioxide removal. Through active awareness of your breathing, mainly when exhaling, you will be able to tone the inspiratory muscles and obtain a better expansion of the thoracic cavity and better lung capacity. Furthermore, respiratory training will allow you to learn how to relax and prepare for labor.

The Stages of Pregnancy

Pregnancy is divided into three stages, corresponding to three trimesters in which many physical and emotional changes occur. After childbirth there is a stage called postpartum, which is a time of adaptation to the newborn and returning to normality. Postpartum represents a new and intense stage.

The First Trimester

It comprises the first 13 weeks. Pregnancy can be calculated from the first day of your last menstrual period. Pregnancy usually lasts 40 weeks.

Physical Changes
In this trimester, a pregnant woman's weight will barely change. The increase is usually between 2 to 4 pounds. By the end of the trimester, the baby will reach about 23 ounces.

Your breasts will change and become more swollen and tender. Nipples may be thickened and have darker areolas. Morning sickness may occur. Starting at week 12 to 13, you will have the urge to urinate more often.

Emotions
Tiredness, morning sickness, and hormonal changes can make the future mother feel tired and irritated. There may also be concern about losing your figure. Many people experience a feeling of happiness mixed with confusion and mood swings.

The Second Trimester

It lasts from week 14 to week 27 of pregnancy. At this stage, you begin to visually notice that you are pregnant.

Physical Changes
Weight gain in this trimester is about 12 pounds. The uterus grows and so does the abdomen, which by the end of the trimester, will be noticeable given its size.

Constipation, indigestion, and heartburn may occur due to the growth of the uterus. In addition, the weight and volume of the belly can cause back pain, leg cramps, and pelvic pressure.

Emotions
Nausea will go away and the future mom has already adapted to her new stage. These are the months where strength is restored and you don't feel so tired. You may feel happier, and you are becoming more aware of the baby that you begin to feel move inside the uterus.

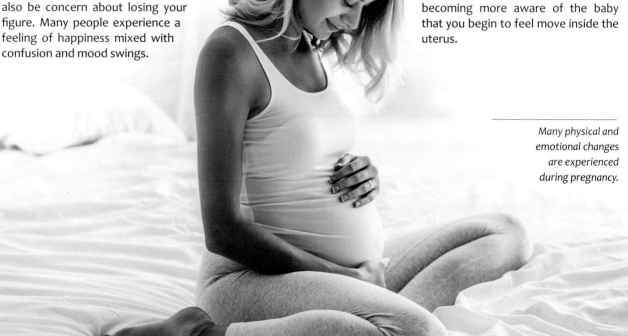

Many physical and emotional changes are experienced during pregnancy.

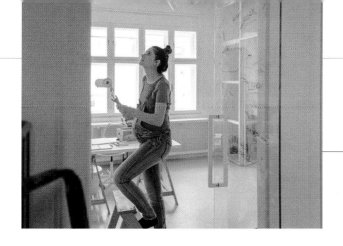

A motherly instinct may appear during the third trimester of pregnancy.

The Third Trimester

It lasts from week 28 to week 40 of pregnancy.

Physical Changes
Weight gain can vary from woman to woman with an average increase between 10 to 12 pounds. Overall, starting from a normal weight, you will have gained between 20 to 33 pounds by the end of pregnancy.

Many women are very well at this stage, although weight gain can produce a feeling of heaviness in the legs. Your breasts will increase considerably in size. Fluid retention may also occur. By week 37, you may experience Braxton Hicks contractions.

Emotions
Fears of childbirth may arise in addition to some concerns about the baby's health. These fears are normal at this late stage of pregnancy. The mom will start to process the separation of her baby who has been in her womb for nine months. However, feelings of joy and excitement of having the baby in your arms will appear.

Postpartum

The six weeks after delivery is called postpartum. It is a period when the body recovers from pregnancy and childbirth to return to its previous state.

Physical Changes
After delivery, the abdomen is flaccid and relaxed, but will recover gradually during the first few weeks. Breastfeeding activates the secretion of the hormone oxytocin, which, in addition to stimulating milk production, encourages the uterus to contract and return to its normal state.
The lining of the uterus will start to disappear in the form of menstruation.

Emotions
There is a great decrease in hormone levels. Feelings of sadness, irritability, depression, and anguish may appear. In the first few days after delivery, make sure to rest and devote yourself entirely to taking care of your baby and yourself. Your partner's help and understanding of those around you will be essential for a rapid recovery.

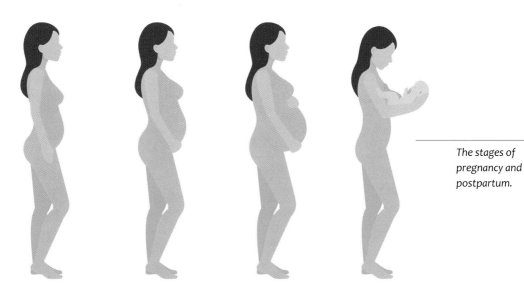

The stages of pregnancy and postpartum.

Fetal Development Guide

Pregnancy usually lasts about 40 weeks. Throughout this time, the baby's development will go through three phases: A pre-embryonic period, which consists of the first three weeks of pregnancy, an embryonic period, covering weeks four to eight, and a fetal period, from week nine till the end of pregnancy.

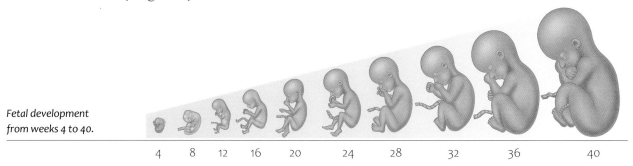

Fetal development from weeks 4 to 40.

4   8   12   16   20   24   28   32   36   40

To calculate the pregnancy time, you normally count the weeks that have passed since the first day of your last menstruation. Keep in mind that the baby will be two weeks less, since fertilization occurs during ovulation. For example, if we are in week 12 of pregnancy, it is most common for the fetus to be only 10 weeks old.

The following describes the development of the baby as the weeks of pregnancy pass.

Weeks 4 to 7

In week four of pregnancy, the embryo (blastocyst) is only two weeks old. It you measure between 0.014 and 0.039 inches.

As the days go by, the brain and the spine begin to develop and, little by little, you can start to see a fragile liver, tiny kidneys, and a tiny heart. This is the beginning of the embryonic period. The heart begins to beat at the end of week five.

By week six, the embryo will look like a tadpole. In this week, the liver and kidneys continue to develop, the neuronal tube closes, and a primitive digestive system begins to form. There is also a tiny outline of what the upper and lower extremities will look like. At the end of this week, the circulatory system is set in motion.

By week seven, the embryo measures between four and five millimeters. This is measured from the crown of the head to the lowest part of the spine. The main organs will complete formation by this week: the liver, kidneys, lungs, heart, intestines, and sexual organs.

Weeks 8 to 11

By week eight of pregnancy, the embryo is in its sixth week of life. It measures between 0.55 and 0.78 inches (spine). Its head is still larger than its body, and you can start to see the eyes, eyelids, nose, mouth, and ears. The arms and legs have lengthened. Some joints have begun to form. The fetus begins to move, although it is not yet noticeable.

Between weeks 9 and 10, the embryo begins to look like a baby. In fact, it is already considered a fetus as it gradually takes on a human form. At the end of week 10, the fingers and toes will be formed. The face has eyes and a nose, and the gums begin to form. Many of its internal organs begin to function and the heart is almost completely developed.

By week 11 of pregnancy, the fetus weighs about 8 grams and measures between 1.73 and 2.36 inches (spine). By the end of this week, the vital organs are developed.

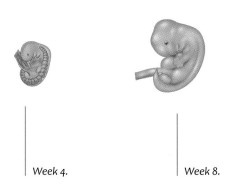

Week 4.   *Week 8.*

During the first trimester of pregnancy, the baby is at a higher risk of harm. To avoid factors that can cause abnormalities, it is important to consult a doctor before using medicines (some are contraindicated in pregnancy), do not consume alcohol, avoid smoking, and avoid exposure to certain diseases, such as rubella.

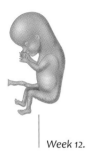

Week 12.

Fetus at nine weeks of pregnancy. The embryo is already taking the form of a baby.

Weeks 12 to 15

At the beginning of **week 12** the fetus, now 10 weeks old, is fully formed! It measures 2.40 inches (spine) and can move its fingers and toes, smile, and even suck its finger. Now it has to grow and its organs will continue to mature and develop little by little.

By **week 13**, the fetus weighs between 0.45 and 0.70 ounces. The liver begins to secrete bile and the pancreas begins to secrete insulin.

By **week 14** of pregnancy, the second trimester begins. The future baby will go from weighing 0.88 ounces at the beginning of the week to doubling its weight in one week. **By week 15,** the nervous system begins to work. Its inner ear continues to be perfected and the eyebrows and hair begin to develop. It also starts to make suction movements. At this stage, its skin is almost transparent. Fine hair called lanugo begins to grow as a protective layer of the baby's future skin.

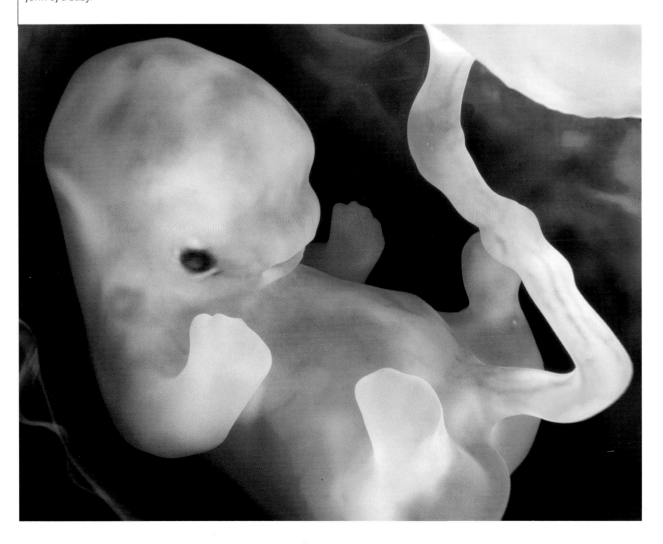

Weeks 16 to 19

By **week 16**, the fetus is 4.25 to 4.56 inches (spine). Its arms and legs are formed and calcium builds up in the bones (ossification process). The future baby is mobile can and coordinate its movements, although they are not yet perceived. The sex of the fetus can be seen by ultrasound in this week.

By **week 17**, the fetus weighs about 3.5 ounces and measures between 4.33 and 4.72 centimeters (spine). The future baby evolves very fast. The accumulation of fat under the skin keeps it warm and nourishes it. It has more and more hair and the fingernails and toenails can be distinguished.

By **week 18**, the alveoli begin to form within the lungs. In these weeks, the fetus begins to move freely in the amniotic fluid. It is usually around weeks 17 and 20 that you can start to notice the movements of the future baby, known as the first fetal movements.

During **week 19**, the nerves begin to get covered with myelin, which increases the speed of nerve impulses. The intestine also begins to produce gastric juices during this week.

Weeks 20 to 23

By **week 20**, the fetus is 18 weeks old. **We are halfway through the pregnancy process.** The fetus is still small as it measures between 5.5 and 6.3 inches (spine) and weighs about 8 ounces. Its senses start to develop during this week. The future baby can hear their mother's voice.

By **week 21**, the baby can swallow and digest amniotic fluid. It weighs about ten ounces.

During **weeks 22 and 23**, the fetus's body is becoming more and more proportionate. Its skin is less transparent, although you can still see blood vessels and bones. The ear becomes increasingly sharp and can distinguish noises coming from outside the uterus. The meconium, the baby's first stool, forms in the intestinal tract. By **week 23**, the fetus weighs about 16 ounces and is about 8.6 inches (spine). The heartbeat can be heard with a stethoscope by this week.

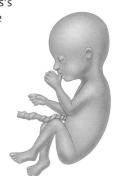

Week 20.

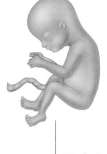

Week 16.

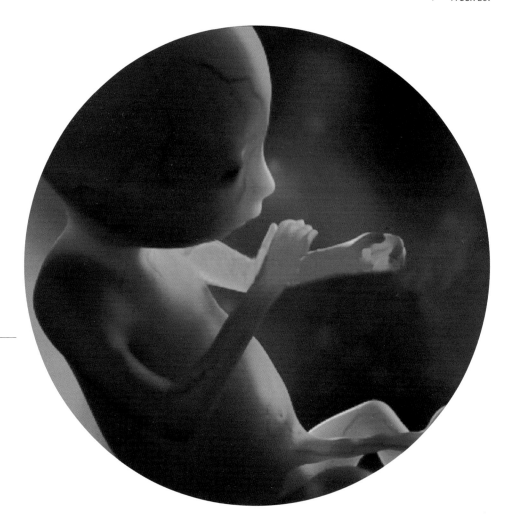

Fetus. Week 16 of pregnancy. Arms and legs are formed. Blood vessels are visible through the skin.

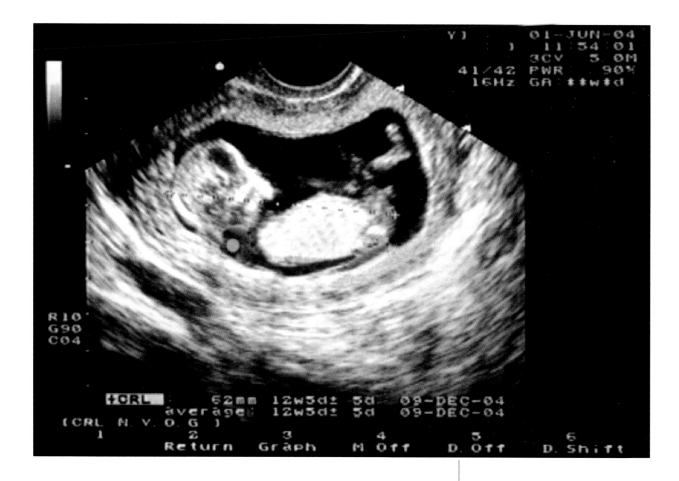

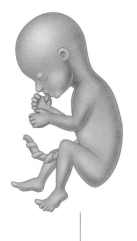

Weeks 24 to 27

During **week 24**, the bone marrow of the fetus begins to make white blood cells. Its lungs have developed but not entirely. If it was born now, there would be a four out of five chance of surviving in a neonatal unit. The fetus weighs about 19 ounces this week.

By **week 25**, the fetus is about 8.6 inches (spine) and weighs about 24 ounces. The lungs continue to develop, the nostrils begin to open, and the nerves around the mouth and lips become more sensitive.

By **week 26** the eyebrows and eyelashes are formed and the eyes develop. The future baby can inhale and exhale. It also reacts to sounds, accelerating its heartbeat and can jump from loud noises. The fetus weighs 32 ounces and measures about 9 inches (spine) this week.

During **week 27**, the future baby can detect changes in light, their retinas begin to form, and they begin to open their eyelids. Taste buds are now active, and one of their best distractions may be sucking their finger. The fetus weighs about 2.20 pounds and measures about 9.4 inches (spine).

Fetal ultrasound is a diagnostic technique using high frequency sound waves that allows us to know the health of the unborn baby.

Week 24.

Weeks 28 to 31

The third trimester of pregnancy begins in **week 28**. The fetus can breathe air and would be able to live if born, but with some difficulty breathing. Muscle tone improves. By the end of this week, it will weigh 2.42 pounds and will measure about 9.8 inches.

During the next two weeks of pregnancy, **weeks 29 and 30**, the fetus will continue to grow rapidly as its brain and lungs mature. Its hair is thicker and its toenails will start to grow. The eyelids will open and it can distinguish between natural and artificial light. The skeleton continues to harden and the head and body become proportionate. By the end of **week 30**, many fetuses position themselves with their head facing down in the uterus. It will be 10.6 inches long (spine) and weighs about 3 pounds.

By **week 31**, the growth of the fetus slows a little compared with the previous weeks. Despite this, it continues to grow and gain weight. Its eyelids open during activity hours and close when resting. It will be about 11 inches long (spine) and weighs about 3.5 pounds.

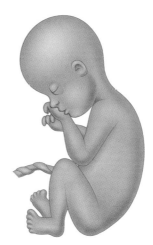

Week 28.

By week 36 of pregnancy, most fetuses are placed head-down in the birth position.

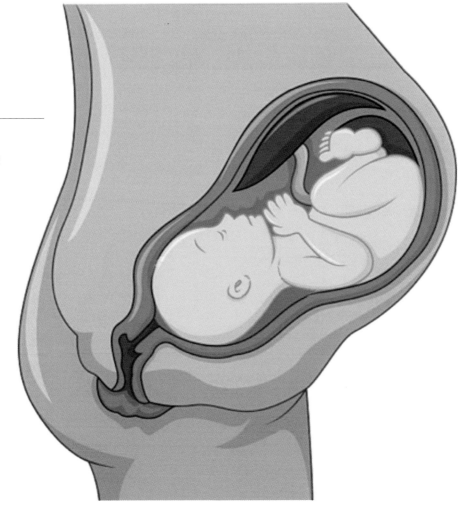

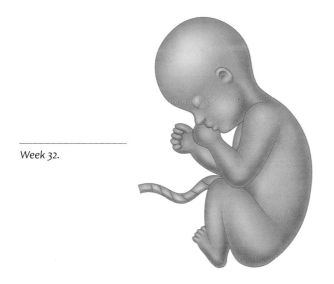

Week 32.

Weeks 32 to 35

By **week 32** of pregnancy, the fetus is now 30 weeks old, weighs 4 pounds, and is about 11.4 inches long (spine). It can move its head from one side to the other and, although it continues to open and close its eyes, sleeps about 90 percent of the time.

During **weeks 33 and 34**, the future baby will be 11.8 to 12.6 inches long and weigh more than 4.4 pounds. It no longer has much space, so its movement is limited. The sensation it now produces in the mother is more of a swinging sensation or dense movement. The mother's activities during the day can influence the level of movement and activity of the fetus.

By **week 35** of pregnancy, the fetus is very well formed. The nervous system, digestive system, and lungs are nearly mature. If the future baby was born this week, it would survive without too many problems.

Weeks 36 to 40

By **week 36** of pregnancy, the fetus weighs about 6 pounds and is about 13.4 inches long (spine). The size of the fetus is already large, so the remaining space in the uterus becomes smaller and smaller. The movements of the fetus will become increasingly energetic, and parts of its body such as the foot or elbow, are more noticeable.

During **weeks 37 and 38**, the fetus is considered to be mature and ready to be born. The lanugo begins to disappear except in the upper arms and shoulders. All its organs are developed, and labor could begin at any moment. Its size is about 13.8 inches long (spine) and weighs between 6.4 and 6.6 pounds.

In **weeks 39 and 40** of pregnancy, the lack of space causes the fetus to secrete hormones that will start childbirth. Its bowels have accumulated material called meconium, which the baby will evacuate before or after delivery.

At the end of pregnancy, the baby's size can vary greatly. It will be about 14.5 to 15 inches long (spine) and its final length, from head to feet, can be about 19 inches. At birth, the baby will have about 300 bones, some of which will fuse until adulthood.

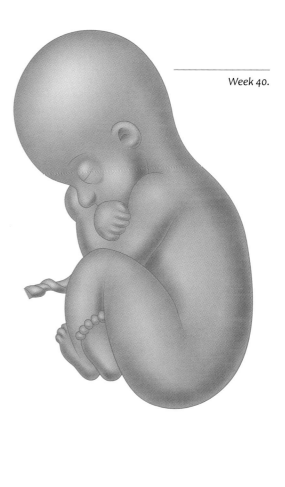

Week 40.

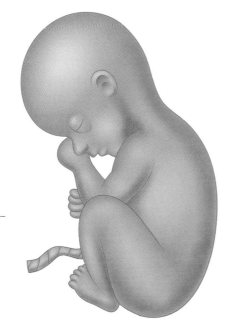

Week 36.

Stretching During Pregnancy

Stretching during pregnancy helps reduce joint pain and improves your physical and mental state.

This chapter explains the anatomical and basic concepts of stretching and how to practice them. The time, area, and equipment needed are discussed as well as how to plan a training session. In addition, correct basic posture is presented for sitting and standing. These positions will be the starting points of some exercises. Proper execution can prevent back, hip, and lumbar pain.

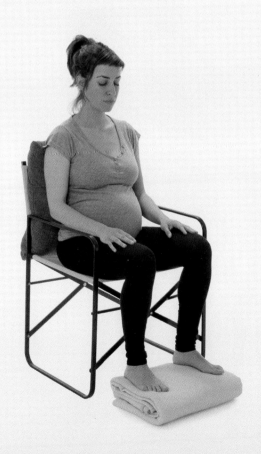

Flexibility and Types of Stretches

Stretches are movements that improve flexibility and provide beneficial results to the muscles and joints. Good flexibility promotes a wider range of motion.

Stretching and Flexibility

A stretch is a movement that can be done anywhere on the body and involves lengthening a muscle beyond its resting position. Frequently performed, it improves muscle flexibility as well as joint mobility range.

Flexibility is the range of motion that can occur in a joint. There are two factors that limit flexibility: internal and external.

Internal factors are those related to the body and its characteristics. The main body factors that influence flexibility are the elasticity of the muscles, tendons, ligaments, and mobility of the joints involved.

Muscle elasticity is the ability of a muscle to return to its initial position after being stretched. The degree of muscle elasticity is what will allow for greater or lesser flexibility. Tendons are bundles of connective tissue that connect muscle to bone. They do not contract but have elastic properties.

Ligaments are bands of fibrous tissue that join two bones together. They have proprioceptive sensitivity so they allow movement but also its restriction if it turns out to be an excessive or forced movement.

The joints are found between two bones and allow mobility between them. Stretching improves joint flexibility due to the increase of extensibility of the muscle.

In addition to body structures, there are other intrinsic factors that limit flexibility, such as gender, age, previous injuries, lifestyle, incorrect postures, or long-standing postural defects.

External factors are external environmental agents. Temperature is the most important factor in increasing flexibility. Muscles and body tissues become more flexible with heat, which is why it is very important to perform warm-up exercises before stretching.

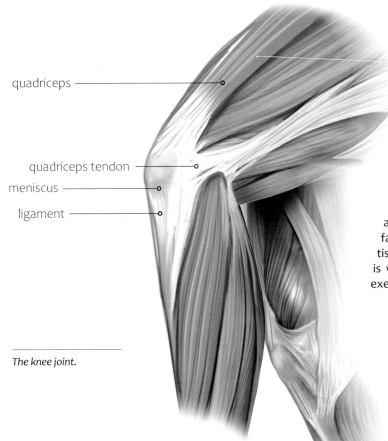

quadriceps

quadriceps tendon

meniscus

ligament

The knee joint.

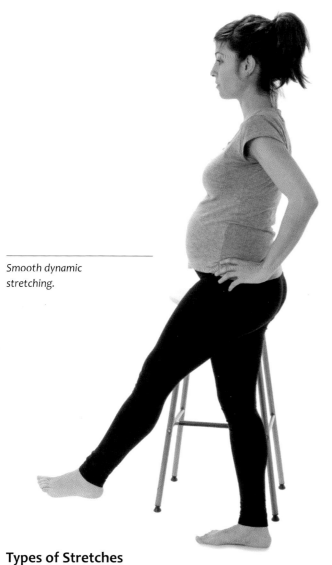

Smooth dynamic stretching.

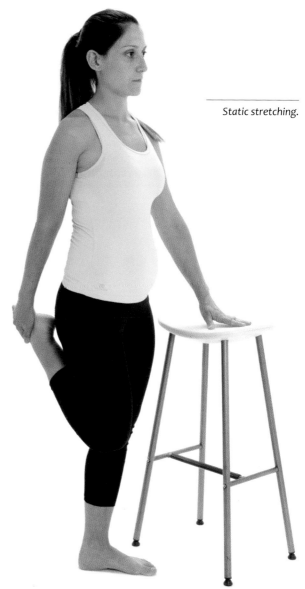

Types of Stretches

There are different types of stretches. In this book, we will discuss passive static stretches and soft dynamic stretches.

Passive static stretches occur when you hold a certain position for a period when you feel muscle tension.

Dynamic stretches are performed through controlled balancing movements. They must be done slowly, allowing the movement to be carried out consciously, continuously, and smoothly. Dynamic stretching will be used in this book to prepare and warm the muscles up for static stretching.

Ballistic stretches are dynamic stretches in which movement is faster and with rebound at the end of the movement. These stretches are contraindicated during pregnancy due to its high risk of injury.

The Practice of Stretching

The practice of stretching will allow you to increase muscle strength, reduce pain in certain areas, and improve flexibility. To do this, it is necessary to practice stretching exercises regularly.

Practice Frequency and Duration

Stretching is recommended once a day, with one or two rest days per week. Training will not be effective if done less than three times a week, and its desired benefits will not be achieved. If you're not used to exercising, 15 to 20 minutes may be enough. It would be ideal for you to combine stretching with some form of gentle exercise or a walk.

Adequate Space

The place should be quiet and at a pleasant temperature to facilitate the range of movement. Avoid getting cold both in static stretches and in relaxation, and keep in mind that maintaining body heat prevents injuries.

The time of day will also influence our practice. You are usually more flexible in the afternoon than in the early morning.

Walking is an exercise that can be included as a warm-up before stretching.

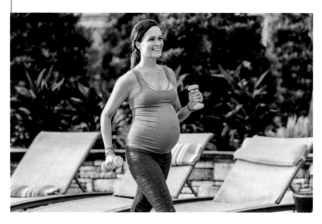

Essential Equipment

For comfortable and correct stretching, it is recommended to have:
* Non-slip mat
* Blankets and cushions
* Firm and stable chair
* Band
* Cork bricks or low stools.

Wear comfortable and lightweight clothing that allows you to move around freely.

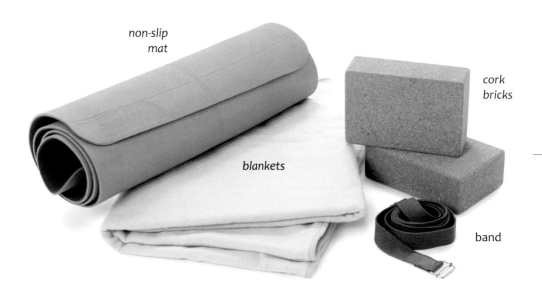

non-slip mat

blankets

cork bricks

band

Basic material for stretching practice.

♦ Do not stretch if you feel tired.

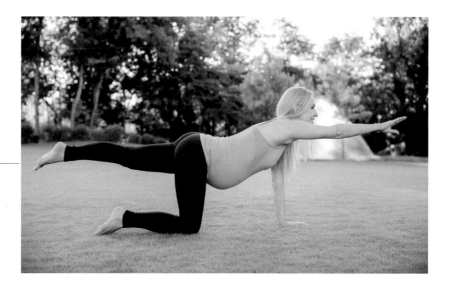

Outdoor stretching is a good option if the weather is nice.

The Stretching Session

Stretching should always be done with warm muscles to avoid injury. Initial warm-up is a must and should last from 10 to 15 minutes and can include gentle exercises, such as walking or riding a stationary bike. Dynamic stretching, such as arm rotation or hip movements, can also be performed.

The recommended order for stretching practice is detailed below:

1. Stretch and Move the Peripheral Joints
To begin with, you can stretch the whole body gently. This allows us to expand our breathing and to become aware of our bodies. This is followed by smooth dynamic movements of the peripheral joints (hands and feet) and head movements.

2. Gentle Dynamic Stretching and Mobilization of Large Joints
Next, we perform dynamic shoulder, hip, and spine movements. Finally, it is advisable to end by slowly walking or moving around.

3. Static Stretching
These should be performed in a certain order and practiced depending on the pregnancy period in which you are in.

Static stretching means more localized work. We begin by stretching one muscle and then moving to the next within the same muscle group.

Stretching must always be done very slowly, and we should never go beyond our limits or feel pain.

4. Breathing Techniques and Muscle Relaxation
To end the stretching session, it is advisable to take a few minutes to relax. It can be accompanied by breathing to release any tension.

Relaxation combined with conscious breathing allows for recovery and reduces any muscle pain. It also helps you connect with the body and reduces stress, relaxing the nervous system and generating a feeling of well-being.

The training plan can be designed according to the needs of each pregnant woman and stage of pregnancy. You can keep a journal describing your personal experiences, feelings, difficulties encountered, and progress made.

The Benefits of Stretching

Stretching combined with some sort of gentle toning exercise helps balance muscle tone avoid imbalances that cause back and muscle pain.

The main benefits of stretching are:
1. Prevention of possible injuries and reduction of muscle fatigue.
2. Decreased muscle overload by reducing muscle aches.
3. Increased range of joint mobility.
4. Improved muscle flexibility and body posture.
5. Mood improvement and nervous system relaxation.
6. Development of body consciousness.

Correct Anatomical Positions

It is important to be aware of our posture when standing or sitting during pregnancy. A correct body position will avoid discomfort and back pain, and will be the starting point for stretching in an appropriate manner.

Sitting Position

Find a chair with back support that provides good hip and lumbar support. To maintain good posture, your back needs to be straight and your buttocks as close as possible to the back of the seat.

Sit in a chair with a backrest with your feet parallel and flat on the floor. If the chair is too high, place something under your feet so your feet rest better on the floor.

Spread your legs at hip level without crossing them to avoid blocking blood circulation.

Your back remains straight. To do this, place your glutes toward the back end of the seat while keeping the back straight. It is important to sit on your sitting bones, distributing your weight equally among them. The pelvis should remain neutral, neither in anteversion nor retroversion.

Shoulders and arms should stay relaxed. Place your hands on your thighs.

Hold this stretch by keeping your head upright. You gaze remains looking to the front.

◆ Being aware of our sedative posture will prevent muscle tension during pregnancy and overloads in postpartum and when breastfeeding.

Shoulders and arms relaxed.

If your feet do not reach the floor, it is necessary to place something underneath them. Doing so raises your knees and favors a straighter back.

Glutes should be on the back end of the seat.

Sit on your sitting bones.

Soles of your feet are over the floor.

Standing Position

The standing position during pregnancy tends to accentuate the lumbar curvature, therefore, we unintentionally shorten the back at the base. This can lead to discomfort and tension throughout the area.

It will be necessary to slightly elongate the lower back when the position in an exercise is standing to counteract lumbar hyperlordosis

When standing, take notice of your feet positioned parallel to the hips. Balance your feet and open your toes in a fan shape. Spread your weight between both feet and move it slightly toward the heels and center of the arches. Knees should be slightly bent.

Tilt the pelvis and lengthen the back and bottom of the spine, slightly lifting the pubic bone.

Imagine a vertical line dividing your body into two halves that starts from the center of your feet and goes up toward the crown of your head. The upper part of the body lengthens, gently lifting the sternum and expanding the chest. Stretch your cervical spine by lengthening your head upward.

Move your shoulders in a circular movement to relax them. Arms and hands hang relaxed and loose on your sides.

⊘

- ◆ A proper standing position helps prevent back, hip, and lumbar pain.

- ◆ Balances the curvature of your spine.

- ◆ Provides greater oxygenation in the lungs.

- ◆ Improves stability.

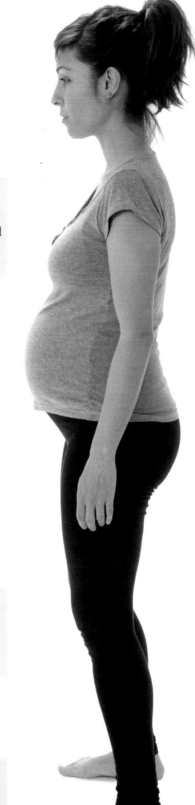

Shoulders are loose downwards and slightly back.

Elongated crown facing upwards.

Knees slightly bent.

Weight evenly distributed between both feet.

Feet parallel to the hips.

Stretching During Pregnancy

M ake sure you perform the stretches correctly to avoid injury. A proper starting position will give us the basis to stretch properly.

Phases of Static Stretching

A correct starting position and an awareness of the stretch to be performed is important. Once in position, begin with slow and gentle movements to stretch the muscle or specific muscle groups. Respect your own limits and stop if you feel pain.

The stretching stages can be divided into four:

1. Starting Position
There are several starting positions at the beginning of a muscle stretch. Many stretches can be performed while sitting; others, in order to unload the back or keep your balance, will be performed with the help of a support.

When starting any muscular work, make sure the starting position is comfortable and stable.

2. Stretching
The muscle we want to work on is stretched slowly. Slight tension should be felt without reaching the sensation of pain. If you stretch too fast or abruptly, you might activate the myotatic reflex and the muscle will contract. However, the muscle will slowly relax and lengthen when stretching.

3. Maintenance of the Stretch
Hold the position for 30 seconds to 2 minutes. Release the stretch and then repeated.

4. Final Phase
Slowly loosen the stretch, avoiding abrupt or unnecessary movements. If necessary, stretch with the opposite side. Change exercises carefully and slowly, moving back to the next starting position.

It is advisable to link similar starting positions, for example, from seated to quadruped, or from lying down to sitting.

Practice Recommendations

The **first trimester** of pregnancy is the most delicate, so it is advisable to always perform very gentle exercises with the doctor's approval. If you haven't practiced physical activity before, you can begin from week twelve of pregnancy. Relaxation and conscious breathing can be practiced at this stage.

During the **second trimester**, it is advisable to work on legs, pelvic floor, body stability, and chest opening. The rectus abdominis will start to separate during pregnancy so avoid any classic abdominal exercises. At this stage, it is important to become aware of your breathing.

During the **third trimester**, it is advisable to perform exercises that move the pelvis. Supine stretching (lying on your back) is not recommended to avoid supine hypotension syndrome, which occurs due to compression of the vena cava.

During the **postpartum period**, it is necessary to reinforce the pelvic floor before recovering your abdominal form. The exercises should be very gentle and conscious the first few days. After several weeks, or once you have been cleared to exercise by a doctor, the exercises will focus on toning the pelvic floor and transverse abdominal muscles, as well as working the pelvic area and lumbar mobility. It is also important to improve upper body movement.

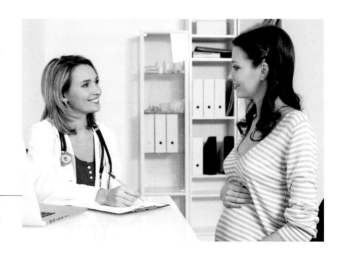

Before you start an exercise program, please consult your physician.

Prohibited Exercises during Pregnancy

During pregnancy, there are a series of exercises that should not be practiced. These are:

- Ballistic or rebound stretches

- Exercises that put pressure on the abdomen or pelvic floor

- Exercises of the abdominal muscles as this can cause contractions and promote separation of the rectus abdominis

- Stretches that expand the lumbar lordosis

- Stretching with the foot in dorsal flexion should be practiced with caution as it may cause of sciatica or aggravate this issue

- Movements that may affect the pubic symphysis should be practiced with caution.

Final Warnings

- The purpose of stretching during pregnancy is to maintain correct body posture, to be strong and agile during childbirth, and to promote postpartum recovery. The objective is not to improve your physical condition.

- Exercises should not be performed if there is a potential health risk, whether associated with pregnancy or not.

- Do not exercise if the temperature and/or the relative humidity of the environment is very high.

- The stretching images are for illustrative purposes. The precision of the stretch performed is what is important. This stretch will focus on the muscle worked on. It doesn't matter if you do the stretch as presented in the book, such as, for instance, holding your foot with your hand. The adaptations are an example of other ways to stretch and position the body in a softer way.

- Always be aware of your internal bodily sensations to carry out the exercises correctly and avoid injuries.

- You should never feel any pain.

- Before starting an exercise program, please consult with a health professional.

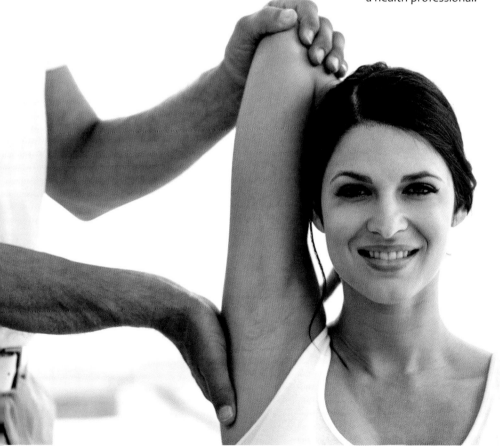

Assisted stretching. One option to learn how to stretch the right way is to have an appointment with a physical therapist. The professional can practice assisted stretching on you and explain the best way to perform self-stretching.

Basic Dynamic Stretching

Practicing mild physical activity has multiple benefits in pregnancy.

The first few pages of this chapter describe basic dynamic movements used to warm up and tone the muscles. Here are different groups of stretches for each trimester of pregnancy. It should be borne in mind that stretching during the first trimester has to be done very gently and should only be practiced if you feel physically able to.

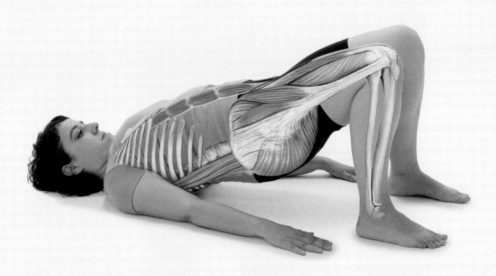

Dynamic Neck Movements

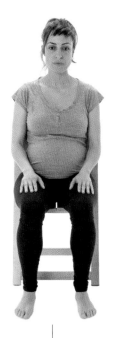

Starting position for dynamic neck movements.

ynamic stretching allows us to prepare our bodies for static stretching positions. With these smooth and fluid movements, we can relieve tension and pain in the cervical area.

Dynamic Flexion and Extension Stretching

Sit in a chair with a back rest in a basic standing position, with your back straight, the soles of your feet resting on the ground, and your shoulders relaxed. Spread your legs slightly and put your hands on your thighs.

Inhale and when exhaling, gently tilt your head downwards. With a new breath, slowly raise your head up.

Again, when exhaling, lower your head by bringing your chin toward your chest and, when taking another breath, slowly raise your head and slightly bring it back. Pay attention to the tip of your nose so that you can observe the movement. The movement is short and smooth at first and gradually expands until the flexion and extension feel comfortable. It should never feel forced. Be careful not to move your shoulders and back.

Repeat the process 6 to 10 times.

Relaxed back and shoulders.

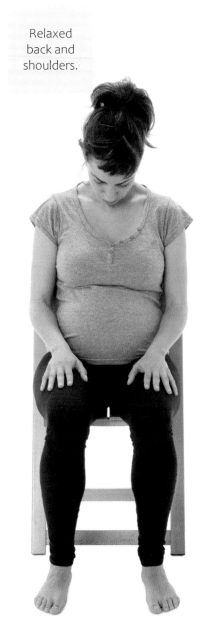

Smooth, continuous movement.

◆ Decreases tension in the cervical spine.

◆ Strengthens neck muscles.

◆ Relaxes the jaw.

⚠

◆ Do not force the movement.

◆ Do not reach maximum extension of the neck.

Dynamic Rotational Stretching

Sit in a chair in the correct position with shoulders relaxed and feet touching the floor. Take a breath in while slowly turning your head a little toward the right. Turn your head to the left while breathing out. Continue breathing with the movement as long as it feels comfortable to you; otherwise, you can breathe freely.

The movement at first is quick, and you will expand the movement slowly until you twist in a comfortable manner.

Focus your attention to the tip of your nose watching how it remains parallel to the ground.

Repeat the process 6 to 10 times.

Avoid lifting your chin.

Do not move your back or shoulders.

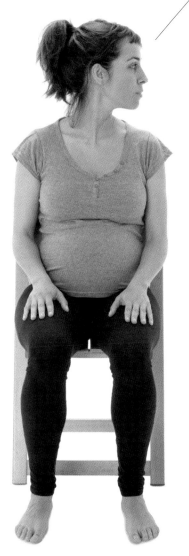

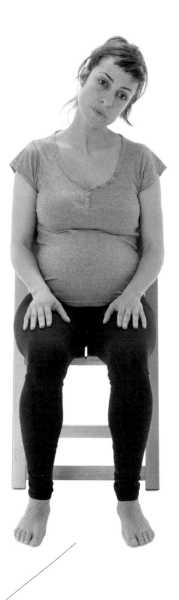

Dynamic Lateral Tilt Stretching

Sitting on a chair with your back relaxed, tilt your head laterally to the right without moving forward or backward. Your ear should be toward your shoulder.

Hold it for a few seconds and bring your head back to the center and continue with tilting it laterally to the left. The tip of the nose acts as the axis of the movement.

Pay attention to not moving your back or shoulders. Do not force the movement.

Repeat the movement from 6 to 10 times with a paused breathing.

Dynamic Hand Movements

These movements strengthen and improve the mobility of the hands. Continue doing these after the dynamic neck movements.

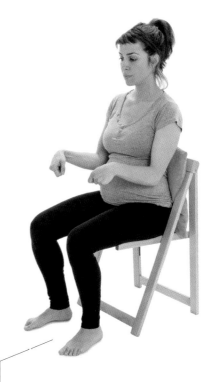

Dynamic Finger Extension and Flexion Stretching

Sit in a chair in the correct position, bend your arms at the elbows, and place your hands in front of you. Your forearms should be slightly away from your body.

Open your hands by spreading your fingers apart and stretching wide. Hold the stretch for a few seconds and slowly close your hands by flexing all your fingers to form a fist. The thumbs of your hands should be on the outside.

You can accompany the movement with your breathing.

Repeat the process 10 times.

Dynamic Wrist Circumduction Stretching

Bend your arms at the elbows that remain at the sides of your body. Place your hands in a fist with your thumbs facing outwards.

Gradually turn your wrists down and out forming a circle. The movement must be broad and continuous. Shoulders stay relaxed.

Repeat 6 to 10 times and do the same in the opposite direction.

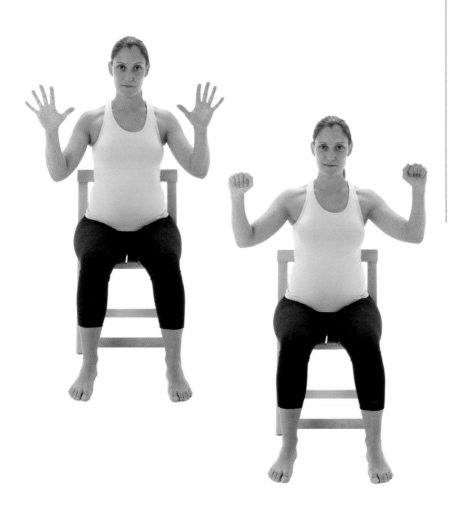

- Improves hand and wrist mobility.

- Strengthens hand muscles.

- Releases tension on forearms and fingers.

Dynamic Foot Movements

These stretches strengthen the ankles and release tension in the lower legs.

Dynamic Plantar and Dorsal Flexion Stretching

Sitting up, raise your right leg and direct the bottom of your foot down with our toes pointed toward the floor. The foot should be pointed (plantar flexion).

Hold for a few seconds and bend the foot with your fingers upward (dorsal flexion) noticing a gentle stretch on your calves. Keep your leg stiff.

Repeat 6 to 10 times.

⚠️
◆ Do not perform dorsal flexion if you have sciatica.

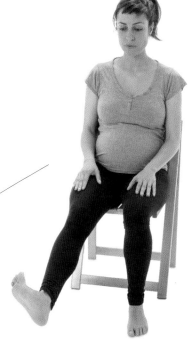

Dynamic Ankle Circumduction Stretching

Sit on a chair and extend your right leg and place your foot in a dorsal flexion. Make slow circles with your foot turning inward. The tip of your foot should make a circumference.

Repeat the sequence 6 to 10 times, and then move on to the other foot.

The legs remain still with the circular movement originating from your ankle.

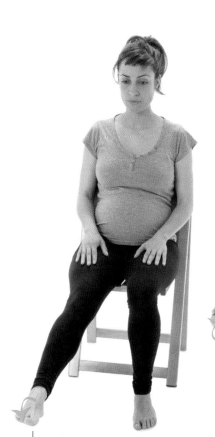

Plantar flexion

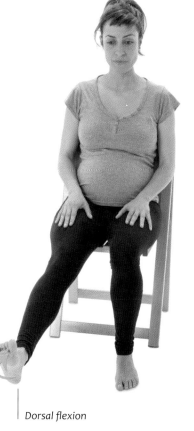

Dorsal flexion

◆ Strengthens your leg muscles.

◆ Strengthens and exercises your ankle joints.

◆ Releases strain on your calves.

Dynamic Shoulder Movements

These dynamic exercises increase range of motion and strengthen the shoulder muscles.

Shoulder Elevation and Decline

Sitting or standing, keep your arms to the sides of your body with your fingers pointing down. Lift both shoulders forward and up, moving them back and down.

Begin this elevation and decline movement softly. Inhale and raise your shoulders in a neutral position, moving them toward your ear. Exhale and slowly lower your shoulders.

Repeat the process 6 to 10 times.

- Improves shoulder mobility.

- Expands lung capacity.

- Expands the rib cage and releases back tension.

Shoulder Circumduction

Place each hand on its respective shoulder and hold it so that your thumb is facing back.

Inhale and bring your elbows up with your arms back in a half-circle.

Exhale and lower your elbows. Place them slightly forward, completing the circumference.

Begin by making small circles and slowly increase the range of the movement.

Repeat 6 to 10 times and change directions.

Dynamic Hip Movements

These movements allow hip stretching and help increase flexibility, improving walking and balance.

Dynamic Leg Stretching: Hip Flexion and Extension

Stand next to a high stool or back of a chair. Place your right hand on the back of the chair and your left hand on your hip.

Notice how you should place both your feet parallel on the ground and place your weight on your left foot. Elevate your right leg straight and forward.

With a slow and fluid movement, bring your leg back, trying not to arch your lumbar spine. Place back to the front.

Repeat the sequence 6 to 10 times and switch sides.

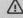
• If you have lower back pain, do not extend your hips (leg backward).

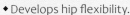

• Develops hip flexibility.

• Strengthens balance and improves walking.

• Relieves hip pain.

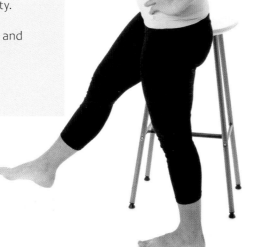

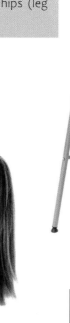

Dynamic Hip Abduction Stretching

Stand in front of a high stool or the back of a chair and place your hands on the chair. Your feet should be placed hip width apart and parallel to each other.

Raise your left leg laterally, hold for a few seconds and return to the center. Repeat the movement slowly 6 to 10 times.

Return to the starting position and perform the exercise with the other leg.

Dynamic Core and Pelvic Movements

These stretches add firmness and stability to your body and tone your back.

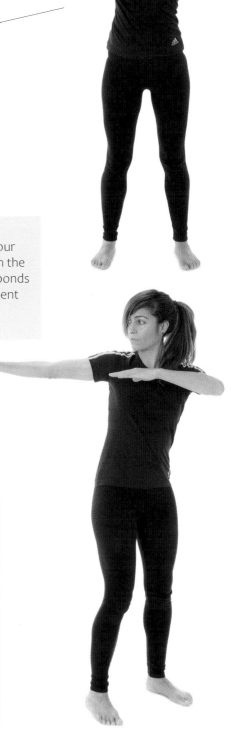

Dynamic Lateral Core Tilt Stretching

Sit on a chair with your legs apart for comfort. Let your hands rest on your hips so that your fingers are pointing forward.

Take a breath in to create space between the chest and the belly. Exhale to slightly contract the buttocks and tilt your body to the side. Hold the stretch for a moment and slowly return to the center.

Tilt your body toward the opposite side. Hold for a few seconds and return to the center. Your glutes should not lose contact with the chair.

Repeat the sequence 6 to 10 times.

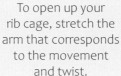

To open up your rib cage, stretch the arm that corresponds to the movement and twist.

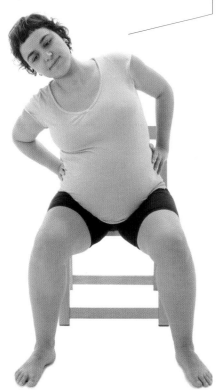

Rotational Dynamic Core Stretching

Standing, raise your arms and cross your forearms together. Your arms should be just below shoulder height and parallel to the floor.

Slowly turn your head, neck, and upper body to the right. Your arms should follow the movement while your feet and hips remain static. Hold the position for a few seconds and return to the starting point.

Next, turn your body to the left. Hold and return to the starting position.

Repeat 6 to 10 times.

Final Warm-Up

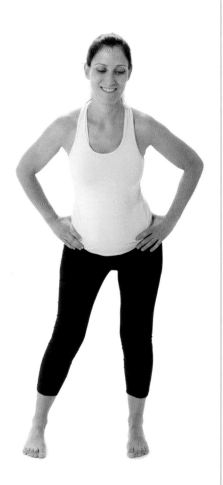

Walking is an exercise that can be practiced until the end of pregnancy. You can walk in place, around the room, or outdoors.

Walking in Place

Stand with feet parallel and hip width apart. Bend your arms at the elbows and place them at your sides. Raise your right leg, which is bent at the knee, while moving your left arm forward and your right arm back.

Go back to your starting position, lift your left leg up as well as your right arm while your left goes back. The movement should be smooth and short. The glutes are active.

Do this walking motion first by walking in place and then by slowly walking around the area.

- Prepares the muscles for stretching and prevents injury.

- Activates the cardiovascular system.

- Improves leg circulation and fluid retention.

- Relieves the feeling of dizziness and general discomfort.

- Walking slowly and consciously helps relieve fatigue and back pain.

Pelvic Circumduction

Place your hands on your hips in a standing position. Place your fingers in the front with your thumbs toward the back.

Slightly bend your legs and make circles with the pelvis by moving it forward, to the side, to the back, and to the other side.

You can also form small, circles of eight with your hip by moving your hip forward.

Move smoothly and slowly. Repeat 6 to 10 times.

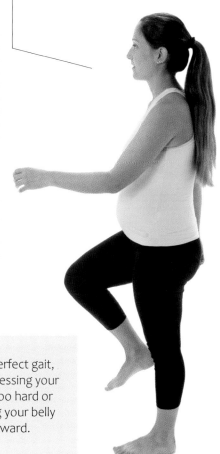

For a perfect gait, avoid pressing your heels too hard or pushing your belly forward.

Elbow Extensor Stretching

This stretch relieves accumulated stress in the back of the arm and helps with breathing stronger.

Sit in a chair or stool with your back straight and your arms to the sides.

Flex your left arm at the elbow behind your back with the palm of your hands facing out. Next, raise your right arm and bend your elbow. Grab your right hand with your left. If there is enough flexibility, the fingers of both your hands will hook together. Extend the stretch by bringing your raised elbow back without pushing the head.

Hold for a few breaths. Release your hands and undo the posture.

Repeat with the opposite side.

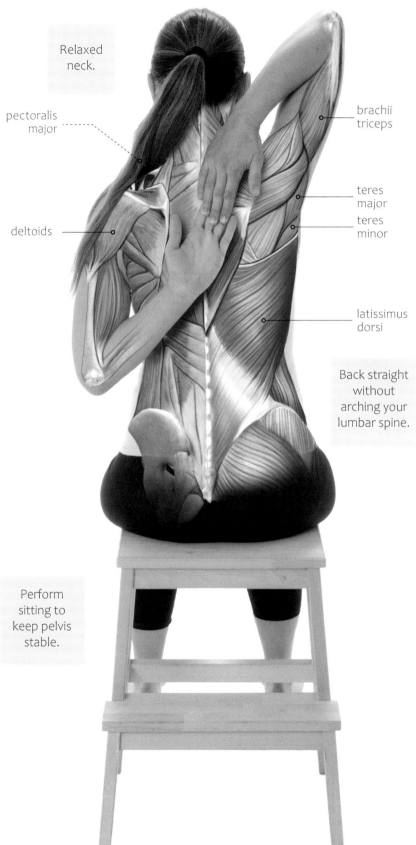

Relaxed neck.

pectoralis major

brachii triceps

teres major

teres minor

deltoids

latissimus dorsi

Back straight without arching your lumbar spine.

Perform sitting to keep pelvis stable.

- Relieves tension on arms and shoulders.

- Improves shoulder mobility.

- Enlarges and improves chest breathing.

- Creates space under the rib cage.

- Respect the stretching limits, if necessary, make changes.

- Do not perform if you are very tired.

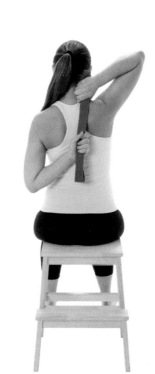

Modifications

If you do not have enough flexibility to reach your fingers, use a band or a rolled towel.

To do so, start the movement as described above. The upper arm passes the band behind your back. The opposite hand grabs the band.

The raised arm will try to pull the elbow back.

Variants

Perform as a warm-up or as an alternative stretch.

Raise your right arm and bend it so that your forearm is placed behind the head. The palm of your right hand is touching the cervical area.

Take your right elbow with your left hand and gently stretch to the left and back. Do not push your head forward.

Hold for a few seconds and do the same on the opposite side.

Chest Stretching

This stretch allows the chest to expand, prevents dorsal hyperkyphosis and improves chest breathing.

Sit in a chair or stool with your back straight and your arms to the sides.

Flex your left arm at the elbow behind your back with the palm of your hands facing out. Next, raise your right arm and bend your elbow. Grab your right hand with your left. If there is enough flexibility, the fingers of both your hands will hook together. Extend the stretch by bringing your raised elbow back without pushing the head.

Hold for a few breaths. Release your hands and undo the posture.

Repeat with the opposite side.

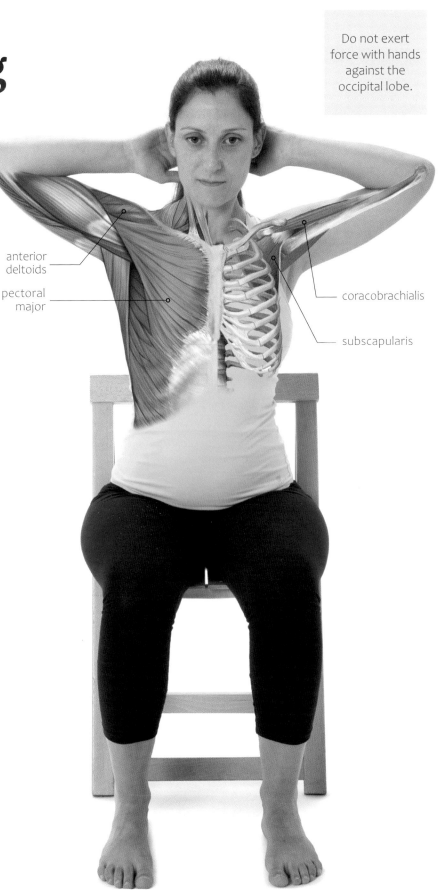

Do not exert force with hands against the occipital lobe.

anterior deltoids

pectoral major

coracobrachialis

subscapularis

Shoulders relaxed.

- Expands the chest, prepares for chest breathing.
- Prevents and helps correct hyperkyphosis.
- Enhances shoulder range of motion.

- Do not exert force with hands on head.
- Avoid stress on shoulders.

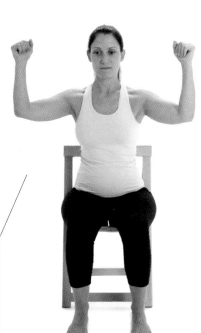

Modifications

Dynamic Pectoral Stretching

You can perform this stretch dynamically along with breathing techniques.

Bend your arms at the elbows with your forearms perpendicular to the floor and arms parallel to the floor. Gently close your hands in the form of a fist.

Take a breath in and open your arms in the form of a candle holder. Breathe out and bring your arms to the center and place your forearms together in front of your body. Repeat 6 to 10 times.

Variants

Supine Position

In a supine position lying down, bend your knees and place the soles of your feet on the floor. Tilt your pelvis slightly so that it rests on the ground.

Neck is in neutral position. Bend your arms at the elbows at the side of your body and place each hand on its corresponding shoulder.

Take a breath in and raise your elbows and arms by moving them up the floor.

Hold the stretch for 20 to 30 seconds.

- Supine exercises during the second and third trimesters may produce supine hypotensive syndrome.

Lateral Core Flexion

Stretching the latissimus dorsi and quadratus lumborum strengthens and tones the waist and shoulders.

Stand with your legs slightly separated. Let your right hand rest on your hip with your thumb pointing back.

Inhale and raise your left arm above your head.

With the next breath in, tilt your head, arm, and torso to the left.

Your body should move evenly without leaning forward or backward. Your neck and head are aligned with the rest of your spine.

Hold for a few seconds and go back to the center when you breathe in.

Repeat the process with the opposite side.

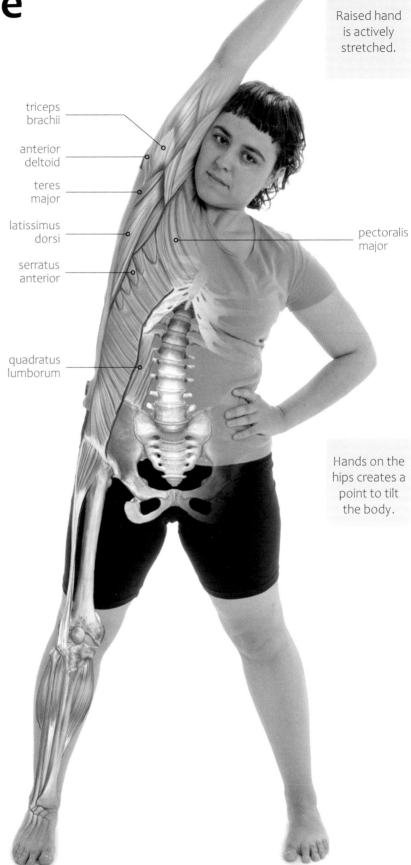

Raised hand is actively stretched.

triceps brachii

anterior deltoid

teres major

latissimus dorsi

serratus anterior

quadratus lumborum

pectoralis major

Hands on the hips creates a point to tilt the body.

Pull hip toward the floor.

- Stretches and aligns the spine.

- Enlarges the rib cage.

- Releases pressure from the abdomen.

- Shoulders and neck must be tension free.

- Perform with caution if there is lumbar or sacral pain.

- Be careful if you have edema in your extremities.

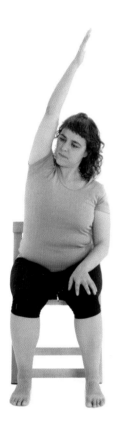

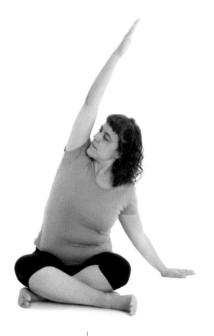

Modifications

Seated flexion in a chair

If there is lumbar tension, it is best to stretch while seated in a chair.

Raise the arm actively and stretch slightly. Notice how the chest expands.

Variants

Seated flexion on the floor

Stretching can be done sitting on the ground with your legs crossed or with the soles of your feet together. In this case, avoid falling back with your body. You can sit on a block if you do. You can turn your head slightly to the stretched side.

Rotational Core Stretching

This movement stretches the oblique muscles of the abdomen, thus improving thoracic spine flexibility.

Sit with your feet on the floor and legs apart with the glutes and hamstrings in contact with the chair and the lumbar spine straight.

Inhale and gently stretch the spine upward, growing from the crown of the head. Exhale and turn your core to the left. Your head should follow your core movement.

Your right hand should look for the outside of your left thigh while your left hand and arm rest on the back of the chair. The hips do not move. Glutes and hamstrings remain firmly on the chair.

Hold this position without force for about 30 seconds and notice how you breathe.

Return to the starting position slowly. Do the same with the opposite side. Repeat the sequence three times.

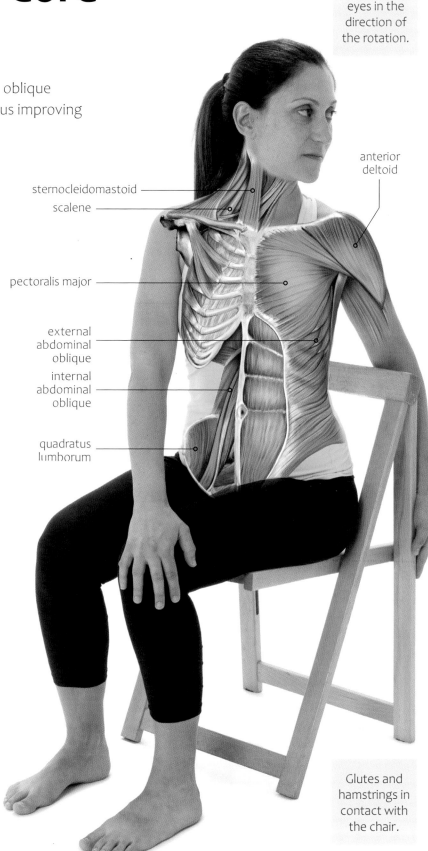

Head and eyes in the direction of the rotation.

anterior deltoid

sternocleidomastoid

scalene

pectoralis major

external abdominal oblique

internal abdominal oblique

quadratus lumborum

Do not rotate your hips.

Glutes and hamstrings in contact with the chair.

- Strengthens the erector muscles of the dorsal spine.

- Strengthens the oblique and transverse abdominals.

- Mobilizes your head, neck, and torso.

- Facilitates chest opening.

⚠

- This exercise should be done slowly and with rotation control to avoid overloading the vertebral discs.

- Do not twist neck excessively.

- Practice with caution if there are problems with the intervertebral discs.

Variants

Hand rotation on shoulders

Place each hand on its corresponding shoulder with the thumbs on the back. Slowly rotate the torso and head to one side, hold for a few seconds, and return to the center. Repeat with the opposite side. It is important that the scapula come closer and bring the elbows back.

Shoulders stay relaxed. The glutes should be touching the chair.

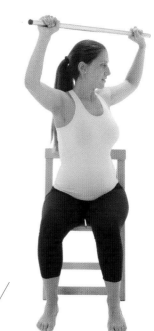

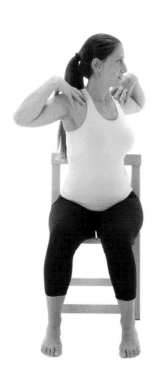

Dynamic twist with cane

Hold a cane with both hands above your head. Rotate slowly to the right. The movement should be short. Go back to the center and rotate to the other side.

You can hold the bar behind or above your head.

Your head and gaze should follow the movement of your torso. Your glutes should be touching the chair.

Posterior Chain Leg Extensor Stretching

This stretch improves leg flexibility and tones the spine.

Sit with your legs bent and glutes outward so you feel your hamstrings touching the ground.

Extend your right leg with the tip of your foot pointing upwards (dorsal flexion). Your left leg and sole of the foot are toward the inside of your right thigh. Stretch your back from the base of the spine upward, creating space between the lower abdomen and your ribs above. Bend your body slowly toward your right leg. Try to keep the lumbar curvature.

Take a breath in and raise your right arm. Place your hand on the corresponding foot. If you're unable to reach your foot, place your hand over your tibia or on your knee. Activate the quadriceps of your stretched leg to allow your hamstrings to relax. Place your left hand on the floor in front of the bent leg. Keep your shoulders relaxed and back stays straight.

Hold this position from 30 seconds to 1 minute. Release the stretch and do it on the opposite side.

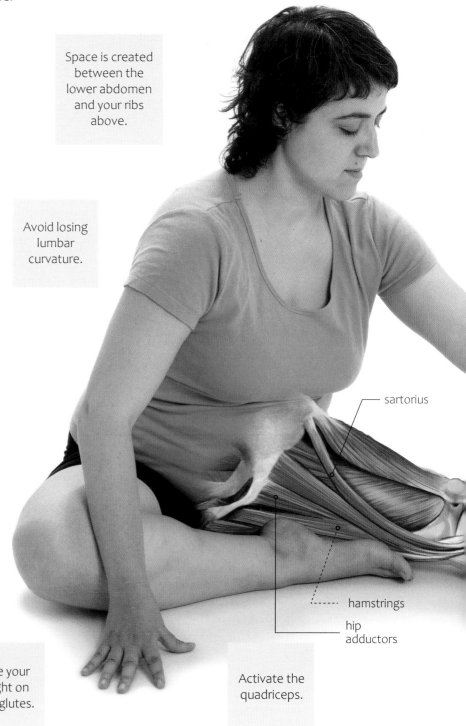

Space is created between the lower abdomen and your ribs above.

Avoid losing lumbar curvature.

sartorius

hamstrings

hip adductors

Place your weight on both glutes.

Activate the quadriceps.

- Stretches and tones the back and posterior leg muscles.

- Reduces swelling in the legs.

- Tones and activates the abdominal organs.

- Creates a pelvic opening.

Modifications

Band and Block Usage

If you feel your back is stiff or shortening of the hamstrings, sit on a blanket or cushion. Use a band to help position yourself better. You can also bend the stretched leg or place a cushion under your knee. Maintain your lumbar curvature.

⚠

- Feet should not be in plantar flexion if sciatica is present. You can perform the same posture with feet in neutral position.

- Place a rolled towel under the knee of the stretched leg to avoid hyperextending the leg.

- It is not recommended if you have sciatica, herniated disc, or lower back pain.

Variants

Advanced position with rotation

This twist variant allows you to create space under the rib cage. To do this, take the outer side of your foot with the corresponding hand and stretch your leg. Place your other hand on the thigh of the folded leg. Inhale and twist your torso and head back slowly. Your gaze should follow your movement. Use a band if you're unable to reach your foot with your hand. You can do this position during any trimester of your pregnancy. If you feel back discomfort or gastric problems, do not practice this posture.

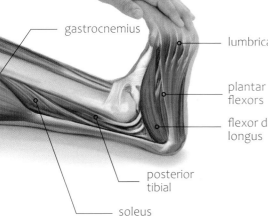

gastrocnemius

lumbricals

plantar flexors

flexor digitorum longus

posterior tibial

soleus

Kneeling Core Extension

This stretch allows chest expansion and relaxation of abdominal muscles. It also promotes wide chest breathing and provides a calming effect on the nervous system.

- Relaxes the abdominal muscles.
- Tones and flexes the spine and shoulders.
- Calms the nervous system.
- You can work the anal sphincter with small contractions in this position. This prevents hemorrhoids.

Place yourself in a quadruped position so that your hands and legs are separated and parallel to each other. Knees aligned with hip and feet stretched in plantar flexion.

Move your hands forward. Bend your arms at the elbows and rest your forearms on the floor so that one is in front of the other.

Slowly lower your body until your forehead rests on your forearms. Avoid arching the lumbar area by keeping your back straight.

Rest for a few minutes observing the chest expansion while calming inhaling and exhaling.

Do not arch the lower back.

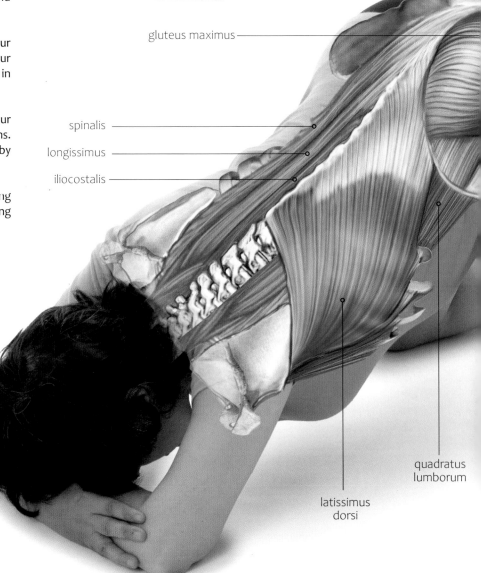

gluteus maximus

spinalis

longissimus

iliocostalis

quadratus lumborum

latissimus dorsi

⚠

- Pain in the lower back or sciatica.

- If you have high blood pressure, the head should be placed higher.

Adaptations

Adjustment of the bench position

If you have gastric problems or high blood pressure, you can adapt the posture by resting your forearms and head on a bench or a chair.

Keep your thighs at a right angle with the floor and your knees at hip level. Breathe and notice how the chest area enlarges. This position can be performed throughout pregnancy.

Dorsal area extension using a blanket or cushions

If you suffer from shoulder or back problems, or from high blood pressure, you can practice the posture with your head and chest placed higher. To do this, place a couple of cushions on the floor. Starting from the quadruped position, move your hands away a little and lower your chest until you are over the cushions. Elbows and forearms should be placed on the floor. The pelvis should not move forward and avoid arching the lower back.

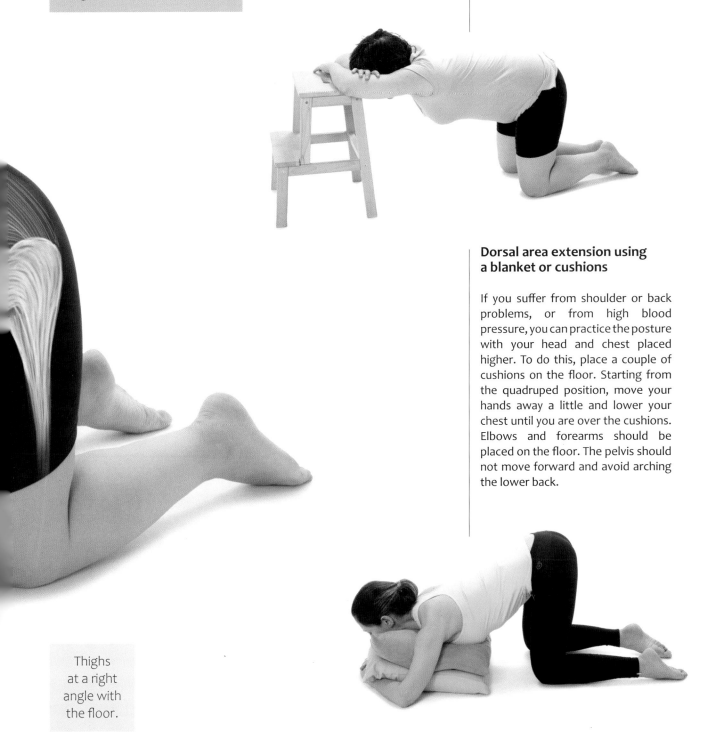

Thighs at a right angle with the floor.

Pelvic Elevation with Hip Extension

This stretch energizes and stretches the pelvic muscles, strengthening and adding greater flexibility to the area.

Stretching in a lying position, bend your legs and hips. Feet parallel, facing the front. Knees and feet aligned. Extend your arms to the sides of your body with the palms of your hands resting on the floor. Slightly move your chin toward your chest to avoid increasing the cervical curvature.

Breathe in. When exhaling, activate the transverse muscle by pushing your belly button into your spine and up and tilting your pelvis in retroversion with your lumbar spine in contact with the floor. Press your feet against the ground and activate your glutes and quadriceps, and when exhaling, raise the pelvis, separating your back from the ground vertebra by vertebra. Do not lift the dorsal area.

Raise your pelvis to a comfortable spot without forcing lumbar curvature. Hold for a few full breaths.

Finally, inhale, and when exhaling, slowly descend the spine, vertebra by vertebra, trying to make the lumbar spine fully resting on the ground in a neutral position. Repeat the stretch three more times.

This stretch can be performed dynamically. When you breathe in, lift up and, when exhaling, lower your pelvis as shown.

- Adds mobility to the pelvis, strengthens muscles and lower back.
- Relaxes the back, distends the cervical vertebrae.
- Strengthens leg and glute muscles.
- Releases tension on the pelvic floor.

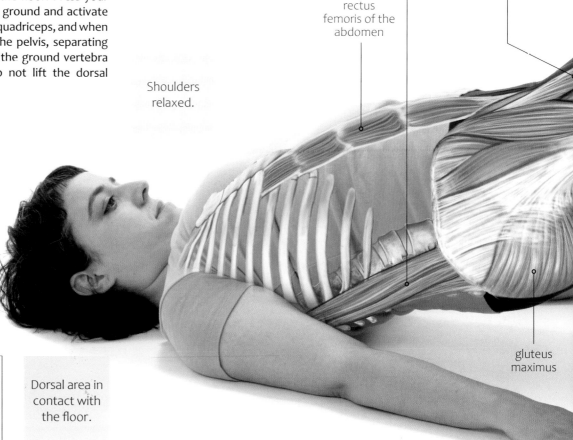

Active glutes and quadriceps.

spine erectors: spinalis, longissimus, iliocostalis

rectus femoris of the quadriceps

rectus femoris of the abdomen

Shoulders relaxed.

gluteus maximus

Dorsal area in contact with the floor.

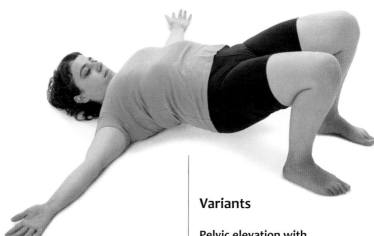

- Do not overload the lumbar spine. Raise your pelvis until you reach a comfortable position.

- Do not practice if suffering from sciatica or hypertension.

Variants

Pelvic elevation with arms extended

Start from the initial position described in the main stretch. Place your arms at shoulder width. Face your palms up. Tilt your pelvis and press your feet against the floor while raising your pelvis and back, vertebra by vertebra. This position also stretches the dorsal spine and facilitates chest expansion.

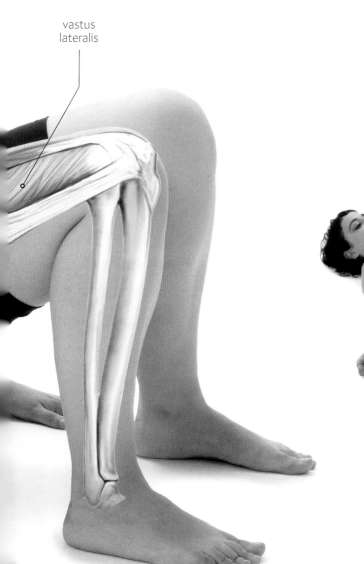

vastus lateralis

Modifications

Supported pelvic elevation

If the stretch is too intense, you can adapt it by placing a firm support under the sacrum, giving support to your lower back. The lumbar area rests and pelvic elevation is shortened.

Chest and Shoulder Stretching

This stretch expands the rib cage and increases shoulder mobility.

Stand next to a wall with a corner so you can hold onto it. Raise your left arm and lower it. Lean on the corner of the wall with your hand. Your hand must be at shoulder width. Take a slight step forward with your right leg. If you want a stronger stretch, you can move the leg opposite to the stretched arm forward.

To intensify the stretch, slightly rotate your body outward as if turning your back to the wall. Do not move your hands and feet.

Hold for 30 seconds relax.

Repeat on the other side.

The higher you rest your arm on the frame, the more intense the stretch will be.

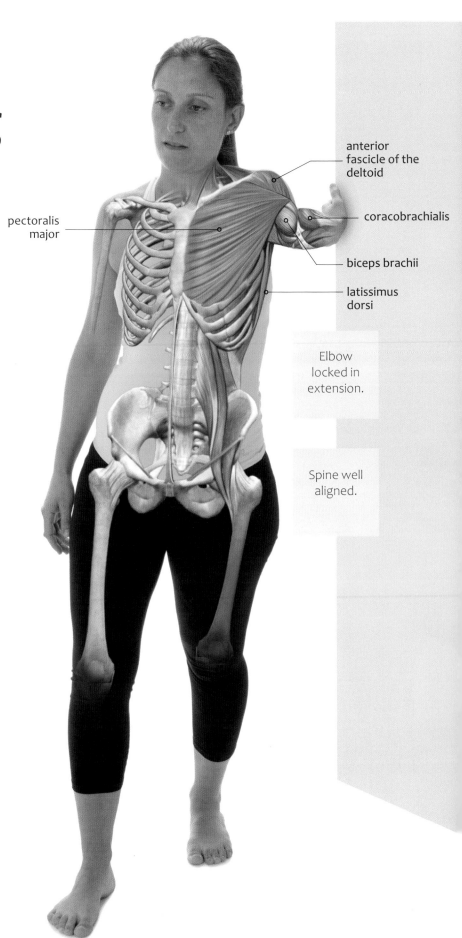

pectoralis major

anterior fascicle of the deltoid

coracobrachialis

biceps brachii

latissimus dorsi

Elbow locked in extension.

Spine well aligned.

- Correction of hyperkyphotic positions.

- Expands the rib cage.

⚠️
- If your shoulders are weak, lower your hand below shoulder height.

- Maintaining standing postures is contraindicated if there is leg edema, varicose veins, possibility of premature labor, or hypotension.

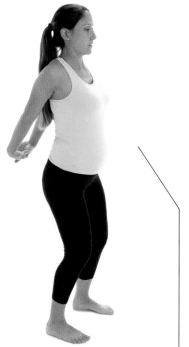

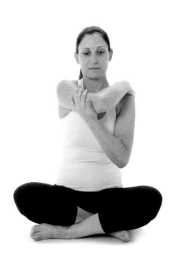

Variants

Stretching with arms back

Place your arms back and bring your hands together so that your fingers are intertwined. Bring your arms up while inhaling. Keep your lumbar area in neutral position. Hold the stretch and see how your rib cage expands. Stretching can be repeated several times. This variant stretches the pectoral muscles, shoulders, elbows, and wrists.

Posterior deltoid stretching

Place your right hand on the left shoulder with your arm parallel to the ground. Take your right elbow with your left hand and slowly pull toward your left shoulder. Shoulders and elbow stay relaxed. Hold this stretch for a few seconds. This stretch improves shoulder mobility and eliminates possible joint discomfort.

Dynamic Strength Exercises: Squats

This exercise strengthens leg and back muscles and provides firmness and stability.

Stand with your feet parallel at hip level and back straight. Raise your arms to shoulder height with the palms of your hands facing each other.

Take a breath in and, as you exhale, slowly bend your knees, and lower your body and hips. Your torso should lean forward slightly. Pay attention to your knees so they do not go over your big toe. Imagine a line that lifts you from your head upwards and counteracts with a slight downward traction from your glutes. Press with your heels, keeping your weight balanced on each foot. Look forward.

Hold the position for a few moments, breathing quietly. Slowly stretch your legs when you inhale. Repeat the process 6 to 10 times.

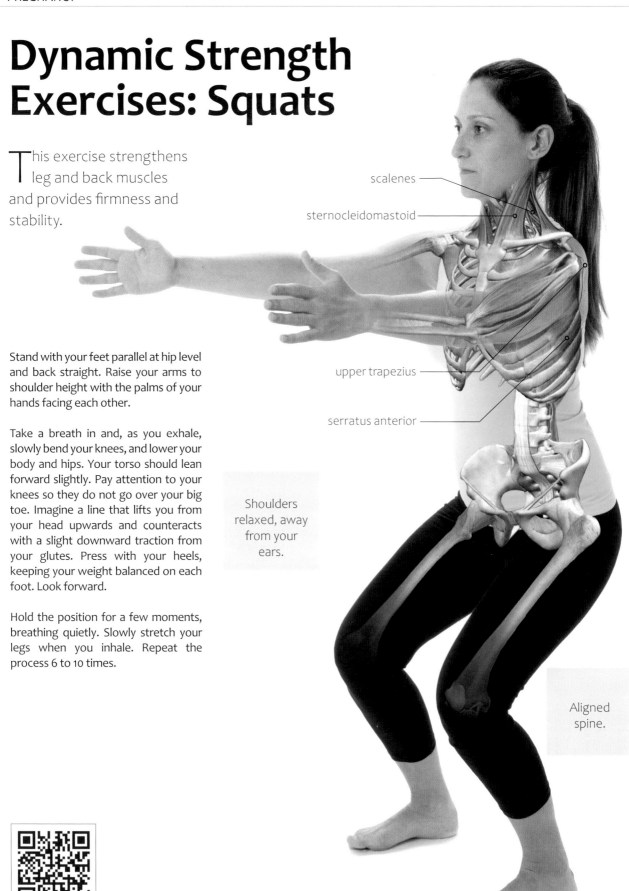

scalenes

sternocleidomastoid

upper trapezius

serratus anterior

Shoulders relaxed, away from your ears.

Aligned spine.

- Strengthens your leg and back muscles.

- Corrects poor leg posture.

- Develops stability and balance.

- Provides inner strength for the time of childbirth.

- It is an intense exercise so do not practice if you feel tired.

- If there is weakness or pain in the knees, poor stability, or sciatica, practice with your back against a wall.

- Maintaining standing postures is contraindicated with leg edema, varicose veins, possibility of premature labor, and hypotension.

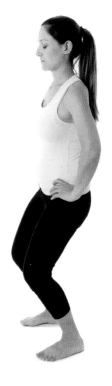

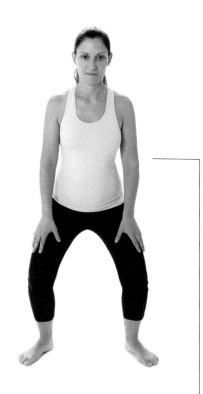

Variant

Sumo squat

Suitable for your third trimester. Spread your legs a little farther than the width of the hips. Knees and feet turn out about 45 degrees.

Place your hands on your thighs while lowering your hips and body. Back stays straight and shoulders back. Keep your big toe connected to the floor. These can be done dynamically or statically.

Adaptation

Hands on waist

This exercise helps us to become aware of the movement of the hips during squats. Place your hands on your waist and perform the squats dynamically while observing how your hips move backward and downward and, when we go up, they move forward and upward, Keeping the back straight. The knee should not go beyond your big toe.

Triceps Surae Stretching

This stretch improves the range of motion of the ankle joint.

Place your hands shoulder width apart and spread across in front of a wall. The right leg should be in front of the other leg and spread about 14 inches apart. Bend your right knee. Your left knee should remain straight. Press your hands against the wall as you move the weight toward the bottom of your left foot that is pressed against the floor.

Hold this position for 20 to 30 seconds and release. Repeat on the other side.

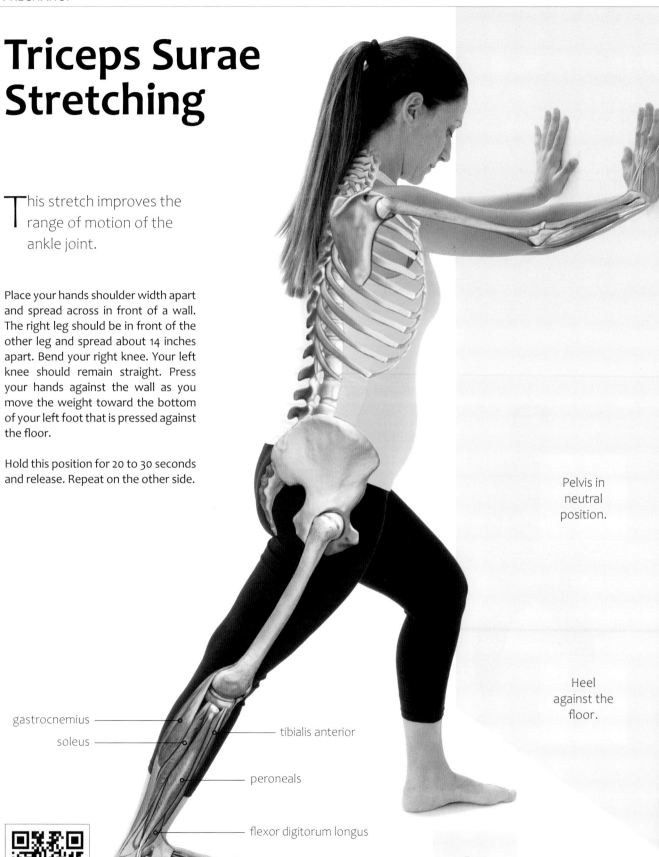

Pelvis in neutral position.

Heel against the floor.

gastrocnemius

soleus

tibialis anterior

peroneals

flexor digitorum longus

Feet aligned.

- Adds flexibility to ankles and calves.

- Improves walking motion.

- Reduces discomfort of the Achilles tendon and relieves pain in the soles of your foot.

- Helps prevent cramps in the gastrocnemius.

- The stretch should not be excessive. If you notice a lot of tension, reduce pressure on the heel of the stretched leg.

- Maintaining standing postures is contraindicated with leg edema, varicose veins, possibility of premature labor, and hypotension.

- Do not practice if you have sciatica.

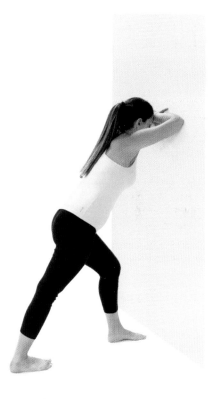

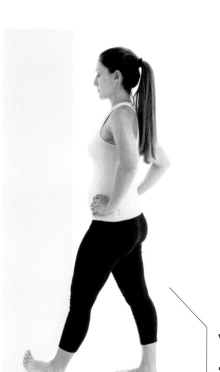

Variant

Stretch with dorsal flexion of the foot

Dorsiflexion stretching can be done by resting the foot on a wall or step. Place your heel on the floor while the toe of the foot rests on the wall. The back leg knee is initially bent and then stretched as your body moves forward. Do not overstretch.

Adaptation

Stretching with forearm support on wall

If you feel discomfort in your wrists when pressing your hands on the wall, practice this stretch by supporting your forearms. Let your forehead rest on your hands. Keep a straight back.

Hamstring and Core Extensor Stretching

Core extension posture releases pelvic floor pressure and stretches the legs and back.

Stand in front of a high table or stool where you can rest your hands. Spread your legs comfortably for the abdomen with knees slightly bent. Feet should be parallel to each other.

Inhale and raise your arms stretching your body upward and leaving space for your abdomen. Slowly lower your body with knees bent until your hands rest on the stool at shoulder width.

Your back should be straight and stretched. You should feel as if pressure was released from your pelvic floor.

Back, head, and arms aligned, parallel to the ground and at right angles with your legs.

Hold the stretch for a few breaths and let go.

This can be repeated several more times.

- Releases tension on the pelvic floor.
- Prevents and corrects hyperkyphosis.
- Stretches the back and posterior leg muscles.

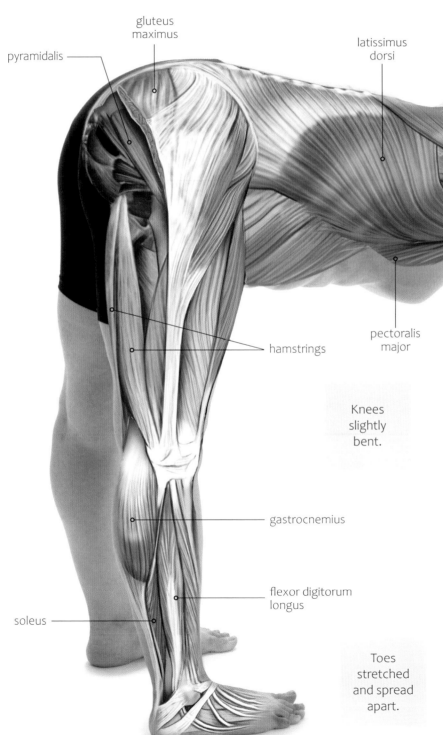

gluteus maximus

pyramidalis

latissimus dorsi

hamstrings

pectoralis major

Knees slightly bent.

gastrocnemius

flexor digitorum longus

soleus

Toes stretched and spread apart.

⚠

- Bend your knees if you feel discomfort in your lower back.

- If you have problems with your shoulder joint, bend your arms or support your forearms.

- Place the stool against a wall to prevent it from moving.

Variant

Variant with raised leg and wall support

For this stretch, use a chair or stool to support the heel of your foot.

Place one hand on your waist and place the other on a fixed structure. Slight tension should be felt in the leg. To increase the stretch, slightly tilt your body forward.

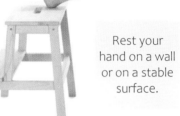

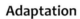

Rest your hand on a wall or on a stable surface.

Anterior portion of the deltoids.

Adaptation

Hamstring stretches with support

To stretch your hamstrings, use a chair. Rest your hands on the seat so that you feel stability. Take a long step forward with your right leg. Lower your core until you feel a stretch. The left leg stays straight or slightly flexed. Hold the stretch for about 30 seconds and do the same on the opposite side. Repeat the stretch a couple of times. Do not practice if you have sciatica.

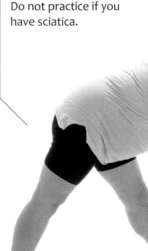

Head aligned with spine.

Femoral Quadriceps Stretching

This stretch decreases leg tension and opens the chest allowing better chest breathing.

Lay on the floor in a quadruped position and stretch to the side in a lateral position on the left side. Bend your left arm and place it on the floor. Rest your head on your left hand.

The lower left leg can be fully stretched and aligned with your body or bent for stability. Bend your right leg, which is at the top, and hold the foot from behind with your corresponding hand.

Slowly pull the foot you are holding until tension is felt in the front of your leg.

Hold this stretch for 20 to 30 seconds while watching your breathing.

Slowly undo the position by bringing the knees toward your abdomen and getting back on four legs.

Do the same on the other side.

◆ Increases the range of motion of the knees.

◆ Expands chest breathing.

◆ Avoid hyperlordosis by keeping the lumbar spine aligned.

◆ Avoid lying on the right laying position for more than three minutes.

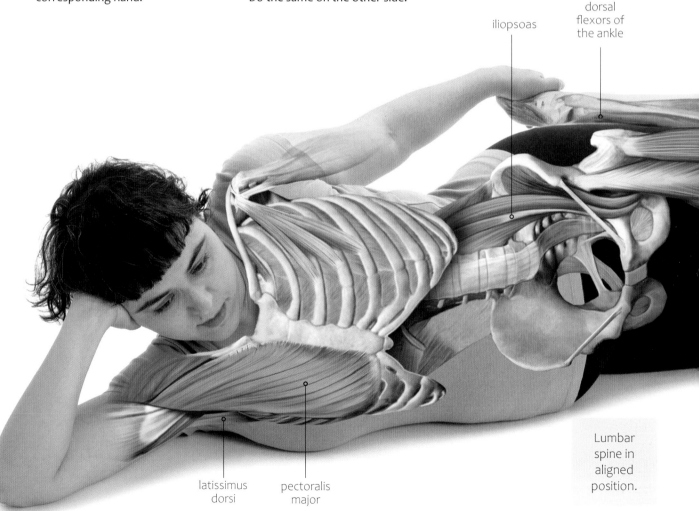

iliopsoas

dorsal flexors of the ankle

latissimus dorsi

pectoralis major

Lumbar spine in aligned position.

Variant

Quadriceps foot stretch

Stand next to a stool, wall, or something you can use to keep your balance. Bend your leg and take your left foot with your left hand. Gently pull the foot that will move toward the glute. Repeat with the opposite side.

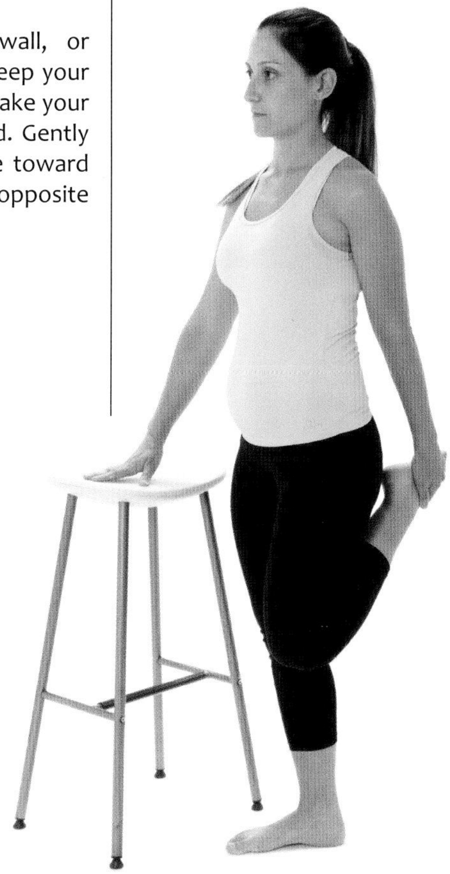

Knees at hip level.

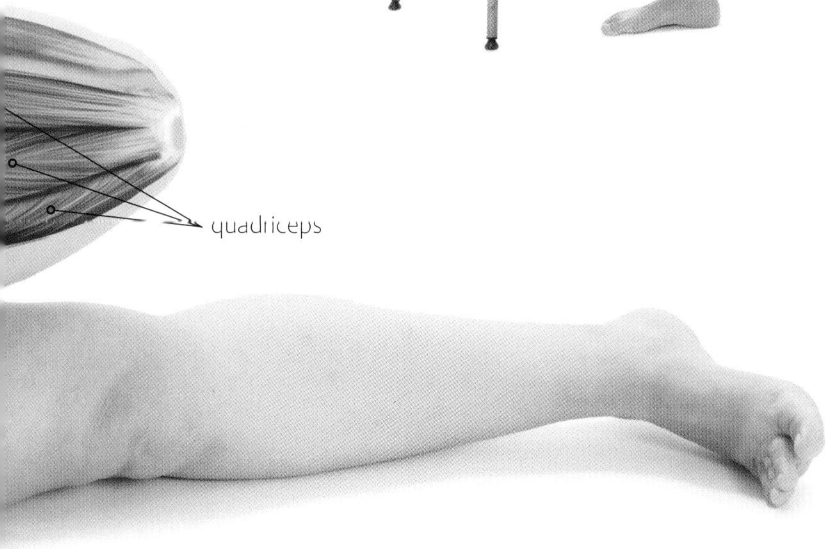

Adaptation

Iliacus psoas stretch

Kneel with your right leg forward. Rest your hands on the bent leg.

Move your body forward, keeping your back straight. Hold the stretch for a few seconds, then undo it by moving back to the knee position and stretch with the opposite side.

It is recommended that you put a thick towel or cushion under your knee to protect it.

⚠

- If you lose your balance, place your hand on the wall or on a fixed structure while stretching.

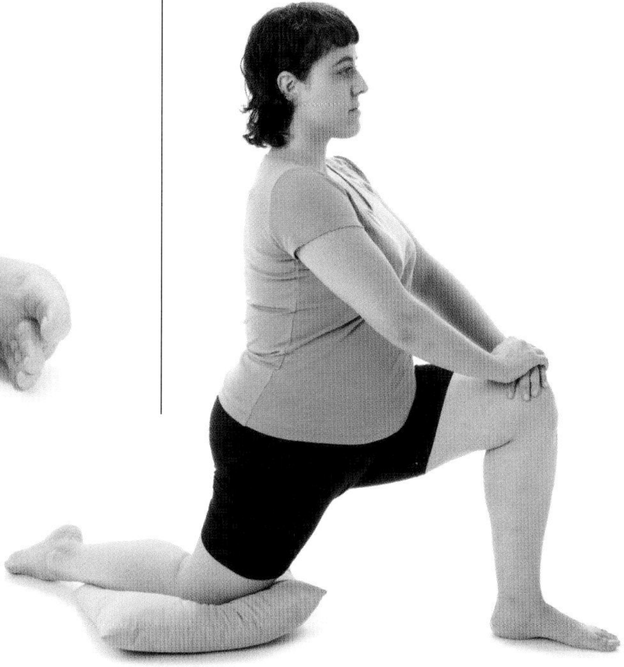

The lumbar curvature remains stable.

Adductor Stretching with Core Flexion

This stretch increases mobility and opens up the pelvis.

Sit on the floor on top of a blanket with your back straight and your legs bent. Notice how your hamstrings rest on the floor. Align your head with your core. Open your legs and stretch them to your side, separating them comfortably. You should not feel any tension. Your feet should be in dorsal flexion aligned with your legs.

Exhale and gently tilt your hips and core forward. Place your hands on your knees or you can place the palms of the hands on the floor with arms parallel in front of your body. If you feel too much tension holding this position, bend your legs.

Hold the position for one minute and release. Repeat it a couple of times.

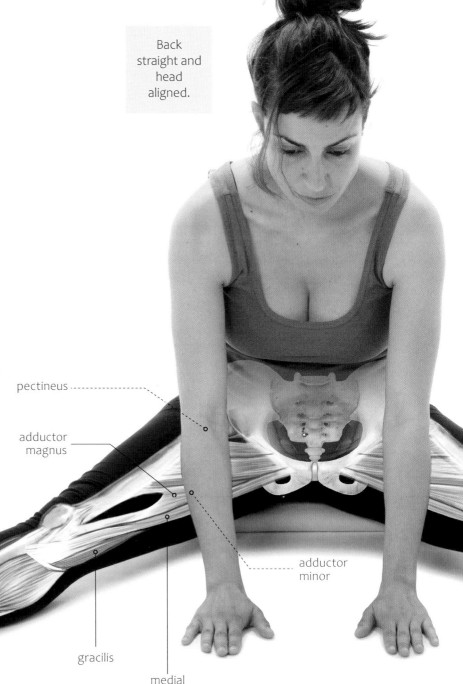

Back straight and head aligned.

pectineus

adductor magnus

adductor minor

gracilis

medial adductor

Hands pressed against the ground.

- Stretches and strengthens the muscles of the back and legs.

- Increases mobility in the pelvis.

⚠

- If there is tension in the lumbar part of the back or lack of flexibility in the legs, sit on your heels or a folded blanket and extend your legs until you stop feeling tension.

- If you have spinal injuries, practice with your legs bent.

- Avoid excessive stretching so that the pubic symphysis does not stretch excessively.

Variants

Posterior muscle stretching with legs bent

This variant can be practiced when you feel tension in the posterior part of the back or lack of flexibility in your hamstring muscles.

Sit on the floor with your legs bent and the heels of your feet resting on the floor. Your back should be straight and your core resting on your sit bones. Place your hands on the corresponding foot.

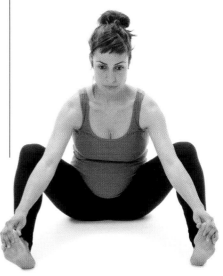

Adductor stretching with support

Deepen the stretch with the help of a chair. Sit on the floor facing the front of the chair. Extend your legs while keeping your elbows on the chair. You can also use your hands to hold the back of the chair.

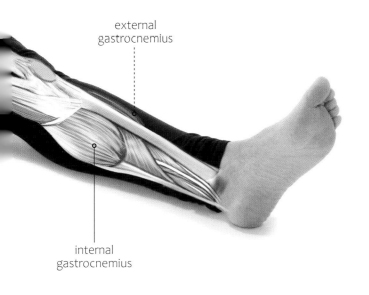

external gastrocnemius

internal gastrocnemius

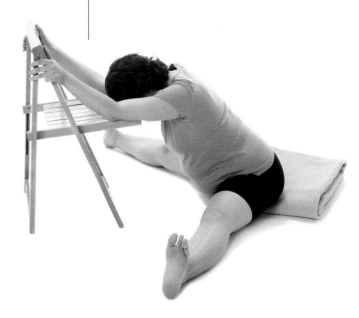

Dynamic Core Stretching (Cat-Cow Pose)

Posture highly recommended for pregnancy and time of delivery.

Start on the ground on all fours. Spread your legs below the hips and place hands shoulder width apart. Hands are pointing forward. Arms and thighs are perpendicular to the floor and feet are in plantar flexion.

Position 1

Exhale, and slowly curve your back using your arms. Begin the movement through the head, then the dorsal region, until you reach the lumbar region. The pelvic floor is activated by bringing your hamstrings close together.

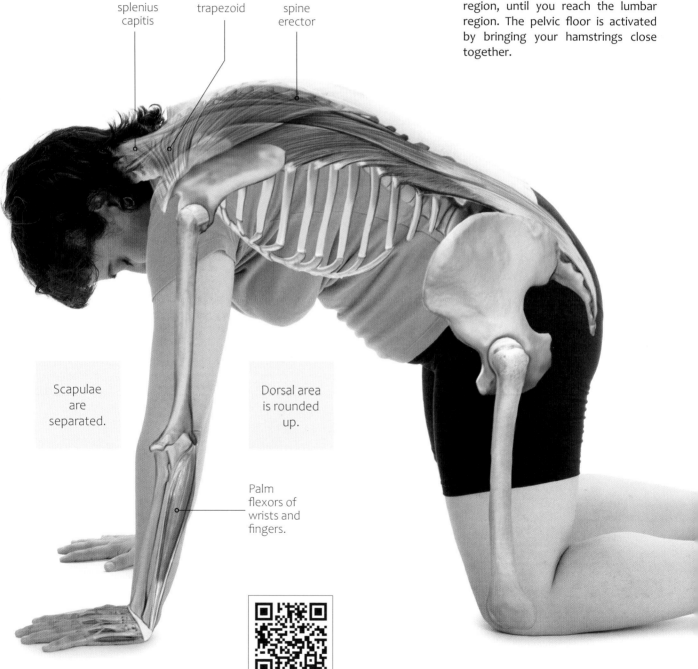

splenius capitis

trapezoid

spine erector

Scapulae are separated.

Dorsal area is rounded up.

Palm flexors of wrists and fingers.

Position 2

Inhale and stretch your back from the coccyx. Raise the chest slightly and align your head with your spine. Do not arch the lumbar region. The pelvic floor is relaxed.

Arms remain stretched and the core should not move forward or backward.

The two positions are alternated according to breathing rhythm. Practice 7 to 10 times, if possible, twice a day.

Expands chest breathing.

◆ Recommended in late labor stage.

◆ It has a calming effect on the nervous system.

◆ Relieves back tension, frees the spine from the baby's weight.

◆ Provides greater flexibility to the spine.

◆ Strengthens back muscles and tones the abdomen.

Back in neutral position, no lumbar arch.

⚠

◆ In position two, do not arch the lumbar spine, and perform the posture while maintaining a neutral neck alignment.

◆ If there is no flexibility in the ankles, practice with fingers resting on the floor (dorsal flexion) or use a cushion under your feet.

Adaptation

Quadruped position with forearms on the floor

If there are problems in the wrists, rest your forearms and hands on the ground and perform the flexion movement described.

From this position, you can work on pelvic floor muscles, which we contract upwards and into the pelvic cavity.

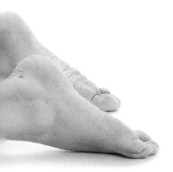

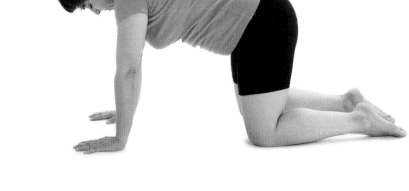

Hip Extensor Stretching

This stretch prevents back pain, allows us to calm the mind and provides introspection.

Your glutes can be supported on the heels by using a pillow.

In a quadruped position, bring your feet together until the big toes touch in plantar flexion. Knees separate allowing the abdomen to be more comfortably seated.

Bend your hips by directing your glutes back and down while your arms are stretched forwards. Place the palms of your hands firmly on the floor. Do not force posture.

The head rests on the floor. Use a pillow to make it more comfortable.

Hold the position for a few minutes, taking quiet breaths and noting the expansion of the rib cage.

To release the stretch, place your glutes on your heels, bend your arms, and place your hands on the floor underneath your shoulders. Slowly rise yourself up with your arms until you are sitting on your knees above your heels.

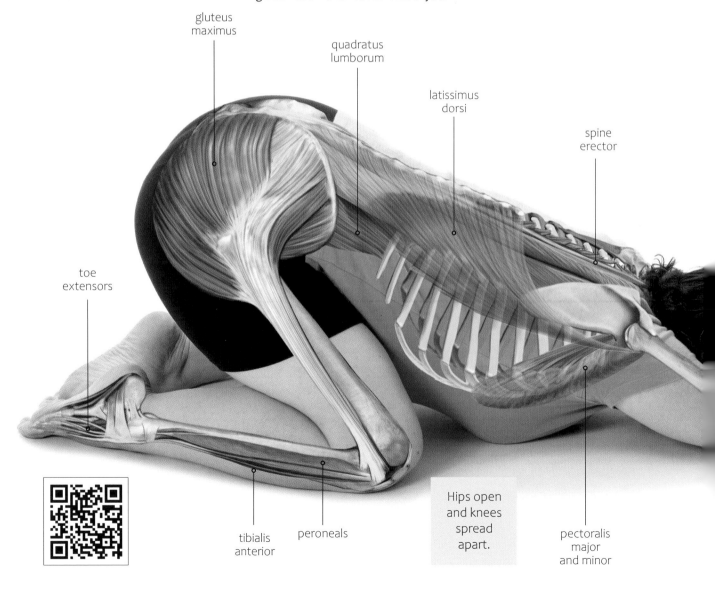

gluteus maximus

quadratus lumborum

latissimus dorsi

spine erector

toe extensors

tibialis anterior

peroneals

Hips open and knees spread apart.

pectoralis major and minor

Adaptation

Resting Posture

If you have a lack of flexibility in your feet or are not able to reach the floor with your head, use folded blankets or cushions to feel more comfortable and relaxed.

If you feel discomfort in your shoulders, bend your arms and rest your forearms on the floor.

- Stretches your shoulders, chest, and upper back.
- It has a calming effect on the mind, eliminates stress and tension.
- Enlarges the rib cage.
- Releases pressure on the pelvic floor.

- Modify if you have high blood pressure.
- If you have shoulder issues, bend your elbows and place your forearms next to your head.

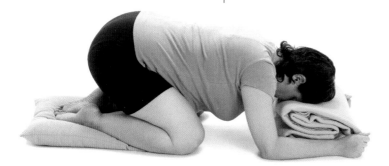

Variant

Supine lumbar stretch

Lay down on the floor and bend your legs with your feet on the floor. Raise your legs and feet and grab each knee with your corresponding hand. Your knees will open depending on how big your abdomen is. Exhale and bring your knees toward you by gently pulling them. Exhale and push your knees away from your body. Your chin moves closer to your chest.

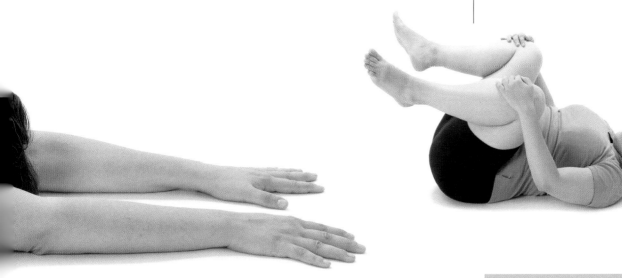

- Contraindications: heartburn or reflux, respiratory distress.

Rotational Spine, Hip, and Core Stretching

This stretch develops spine mobility and opens the chest making breathing easier. It also induces a calm state of mind.

In a quadruped position, stretch sideways to the right in a lateral position. Bend your knees and place a pillow between both legs. Stretch your arms at shoulder width by bringing the palms of your hands together. Pay close attention to the correct position of your shoulders, knees, and feet, which must be aligned with each other.

Inhale and raise your arm upwards. Raise your head toward the arm facing upwards. If you are flexible enough, lower your arm until it rests on the floor behind your back. Tilt your head in the same direction.

Hold this position statically for a few minutes or alternate with dynamic arm movements. Repeat with the opposite side.

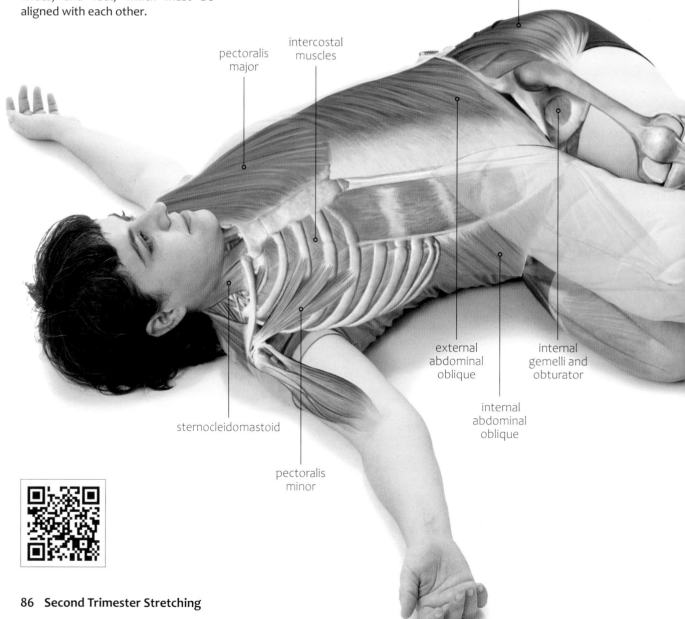

gluteus

intercostal muscles

pectoralis major

external abdominal oblique

internal gemelli and obturator

internal abdominal oblique

sternocleidomastoid

pectoralis minor

- Opens the chest and makes breathing easier.

- Brings mobility to the spine.

- Stimulates and tones the spinal nerves, relaxing the nervous system.

- Back pain, acute sciatica, or herniated discs.

- If you have lumbar problems, practice with caution and in a sedative position.

- Do not maintain posture for more than three minutes to avoid supine hypotensive syndrome.

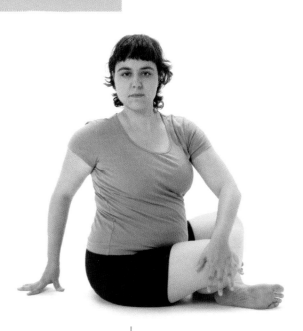

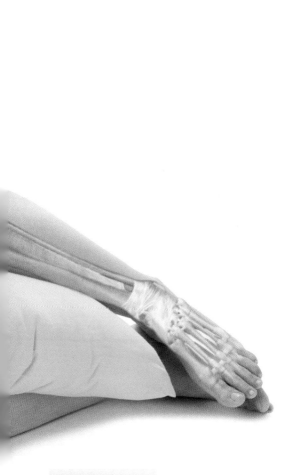

Place a pillow under your arm (left) to avoid forcing rotation.

Variant

Torsion in a sedative position

Cross your legs on the floor. Grab your right knee with your left hand while twisting your body with your right hand by placing it behind your back. Your head should rotate with your body. Your glutes are on the floor and shoulders are at the same height.

Posterior Chain Stretching with Legs Raised

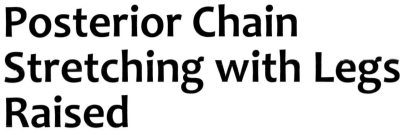

This stretch improves leg circulation and relaxation in the sacrum and lower back.

Sit on the floor near a wall. Stretch in a lateral position bringing your glutes as close as possible toward the wall. Stretch your body on the floor and raise your legs vertically by stretching them and resting them on the wall. Make sure your body, legs, and head are aligned. Knees should stay slightly bent. Arms are extended on both sides and relaxed.

Hold this stretch for a few minutes while breathing calmly.

To release, bend your legs toward your body and rotate to the left side until you are back in a lateral position.

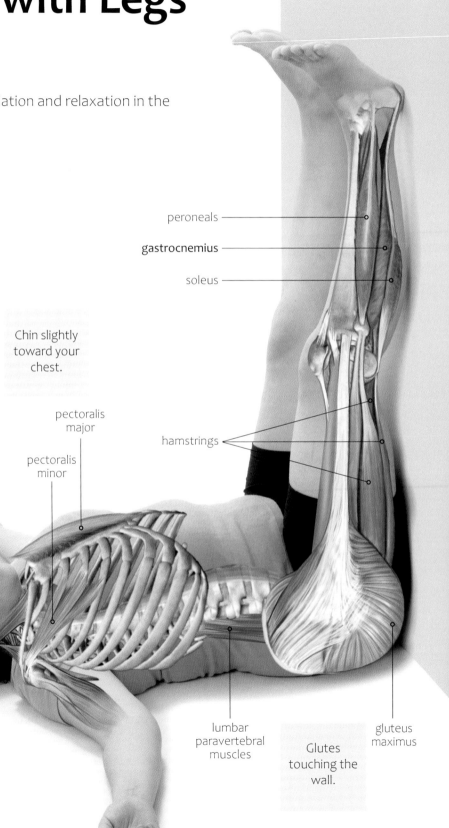

Chin slightly toward your chest.

peroneals

gastrocnemius

soleus

hamstrings

pectoralis major

pectoralis minor

lumbar paravertebral muscles

Glutes touching the wall.

gluteus maximus

Arms relaxed.

♦ Improvement of blood circulation and venous return in legs and pelvis, relieving varicose veins and hemorrhoids.

♦ Relaxes the sacrum and lumbar spine.

⚠

♦ The cervical spine is stretched without hyperextension.

♦ Prolonged supine position from the second and third trimester of pregnancy should be avoided to avoid supine hypotensive syndrome.

Variants

Posterior chain and adductor stretching

Begin by separating your legs on both sides. Spread your legs apart until you feel the stretch but in a comfortable manner. Keep your head and neck relaxed. If necessary, use pillows under your head.

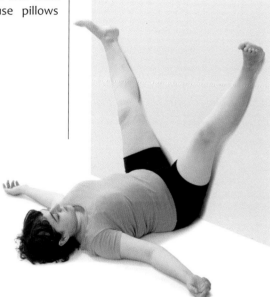

Rest position

Bend your legs like a butterfly and try to bring the soles of your feet close together. Rest your feet on the wall. Place a pillow under your head. This position helps to open the pelvis and helps your pelvic floor rest.

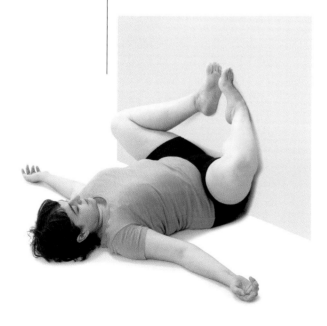

Core Stretching

This posture revitalizes the body and tones your back muscles.

Sit on the floor cross-legged with your right foot placed under the left leg. Pelvis and back are in neutral position. Stretch from your head up.

Inhale and raise your arms up above your head. Arms are shoulder width apart. Stretch your hands with palms facing each other and extending your fingers up. Back is straight, avoid tilting your body backward. Hold the position without tensing your shoulder so that they are far from your ears. Face and neck are relaxed. Notice how there is space in the abdomen when you lift your body and how it favors thoracic breathing.

Hold this position for a few complete breaths and release. Repeat the stretch by alternating your legs.

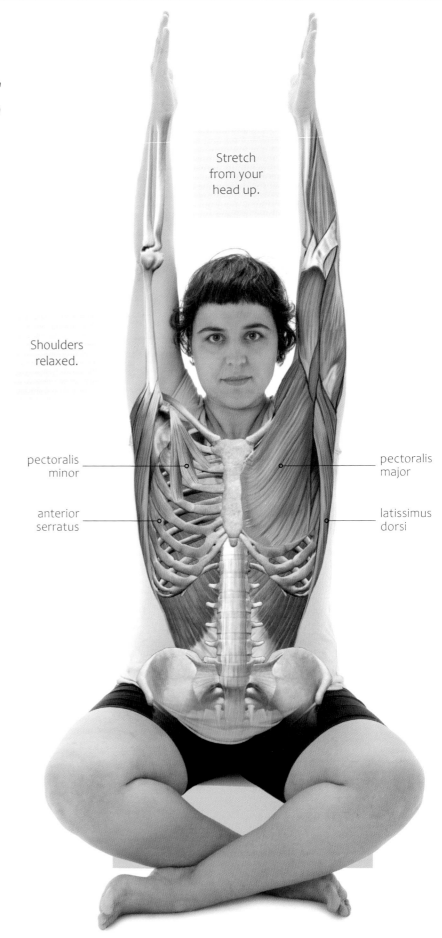

Stretch from your head up.

Shoulders relaxed.

pectoralis minor

anterior serratus

pectoralis major

latissimus dorsi

Sit on your glutes and hamstrings.

- Tones and strengthens back and arm muscles.
- Revitalizes the body.
- Stretches your back and expands your chest.

- If shoulder pain occurs, do not fully stretch your arms upwards, but lift them in front of your head.

Variants

Upper core stretching with hands together

This variant, with your hands held together by the thumb, may be more comfortable.

Begin in the main position. Stretch your arms and join your hands by intertwining your thumbs with palms facing the front. Hold this position for a few breaths and release.

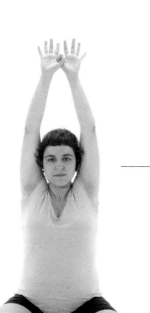

Dorsal stretching with finger extension

Stand or sit in a chair. Interlace your fingers and stretch your arms over your head. Turn your wrists so that the palms of your hands are facing up. Make sure your pelvis remains neutral. Hold this position for 10 to 15 seconds, breathing quietly. Repeat by changing your interlaced fingers. Do not force the position of your hands.

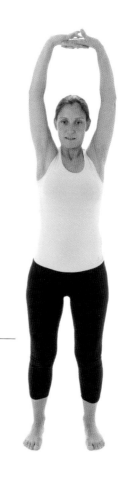

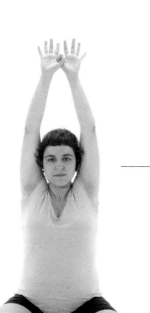

Isometric Chest Contractions

These movements strengthen the pectoral muscles, the biceps brachii, and the triceps.

Only the chest stretches, the rest of your body remains relaxed.

Sit with your back straight and feet flat on the floor parallel to each other. Bend your elbows and bring the palms of your hands together in front of your chest. Place your arms slightly below the shoulders.

Perform a thoracic inhalation and, when exhaling slowly, contract the abdomen and press the palms of your hands against each other. Hold the contraction for a few seconds, breathing normally, and relax.

Repeat the sequence 6 to 10 times.

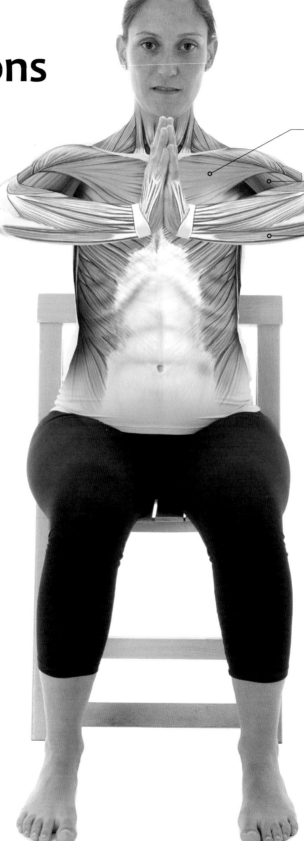

Do not hold your breath.

pectoralis minor

biceps brachii

flexor digitorum profundus

Shoulders relaxed.

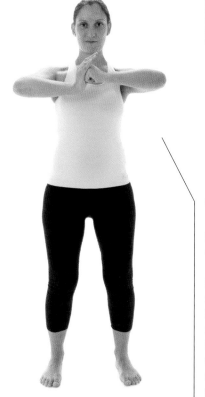

✓
• Tones and strengthens chest muscles.

⚠
• This isometric work should only be held for a few seconds.

• Failure to breathe throughout may increase intra-abdominal pressure.

• Hypertension.

Variantes

Isometric contractions with Closed Fist

Bend your arms at the elbows and raise them just below shoulder height. Place your left hand in the form of a fist and place your right palm over it. Exhale, contract the transversus abdominis and press your hands one against the other, holding the pressure for a few seconds while breathing normally. Release. Repeat the sequence 6 to 10 times.

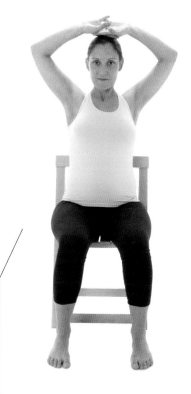

Isometric contractions with upward finger and arm extension

Raise your arms with your elbows bent. Place the back of your hands above your head. Interlace your hand fingers and rotate your wrists so that the palms of your hands face upwards. Press your hands for a second as if you were to push your hands together more and relax. Repeat 6 to 10 times.

Thoracic Spine Extension

This extension relieves discomfort in the thoracic spine and improves chest breathing.

Sit with a straight back and glutes firmly on the chair. Place a pillow on the back of the chair. Spread your legs a little wider than the width of your hips. Feet rest on the floor. Knees aligned with feet. The head in line with the spine. Face front.

Inhale and bring your arms back without raising your shoulders. Hold the back of the seat with your hands. Shoulder blades come together slightly. Lift your chest from the sternum. The pelvis is supported without moving forward. Do not accentuate the lumbar curve of the back (hyperlordosis).

Hold for a few minutes breathing quietly and watch how your ribs and thorax expand.

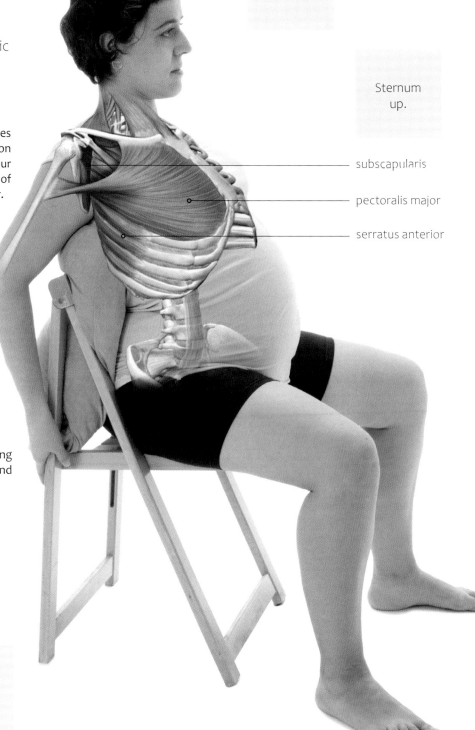

Face forward.

Sternum up.

subscapularis

pectoralis major

serratus anterior

Pelvis properly supported.

- Increases chest breathing by increasing breathing capacity.

- Increases awareness of breathing.

- Prevents and corrects hyperkyphosis.

- Relieves discomfort in the dorsal spine.

- Do not hyperextend the lumbar spine.

- Do not perform this exercise too vigorously as it can injure your shoulders.

Variants

Core extension on the floor with support

This posture stretches the posterior part of your legs. Sit on the floor with your legs apart and back resting on the seat. Place your arms back and hold the front legs of the chair with your hands to support your dorsal muscles and expand the rib cage.

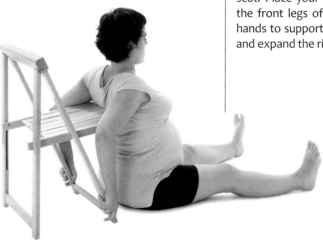

Advanced core extension

This position strengthens the back muscles and stretches the muscles on the back of your legs. To perform this posture, we suggest placing a pillow under your coccyx to raise the pelvis. Press the floor with your hands and push your breastbone upwards. Do not perform if you feel tired, have heart problems, or if there are spinal injuries.

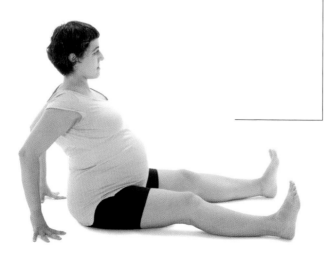

Thoracic Spine Extension 95

Gluteus Maximus Strength Work

In this posture, you can tone and strengthen your glutes as well as work on stabilizing the spine and pelvis.

On all fours with your legs spread hip width apart and arms and hands under their corresponding shoulder.

Inhale and activate your glutes, exhale, and raise your leg off the floor. This should not go past the height of your hips. The pelvis and core remain in place and firm.

Hold for two breaths and release. Repeat three more times.

Perform the position with the opposite leg.

- Glute strengthening.
- Promotes stability and balance.

  Strengthens your arms.

- The spine must not arch forward.
- Avoid hyperlordosis.
- Place a pillow to support your knees.

Raise your leg up to the height of your hips to avoid overloading your lower back.

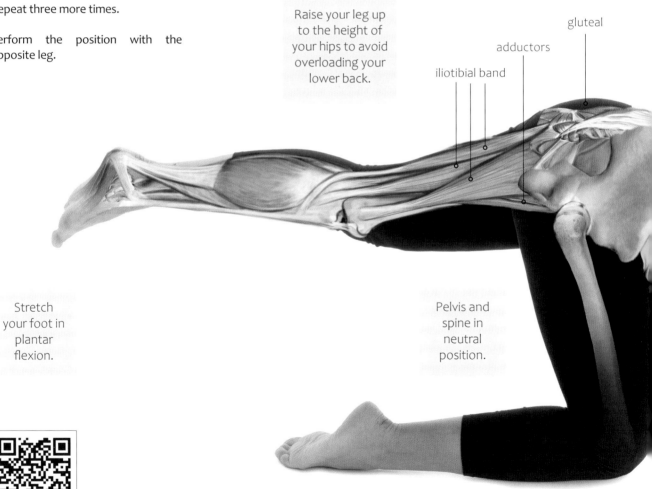

iliotibial band

adductors

gluteal

Stretch your foot in plantar flexion.

Pelvis and spine in neutral position.

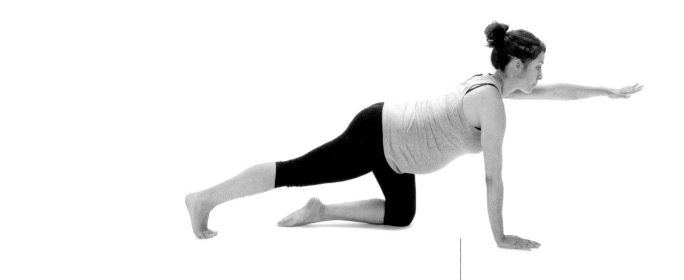

Variant

Stance with arm raised

Begin from the previous position. Stretch one leg back with your foot resting on the floor while lifting the opposite arm. If you want to extend the exercise, exhale, and raise the straightened leg. Hold for one breath and, when exhaling, return to the starting position. Repeat on the opposite side.

spine erector · multifidus

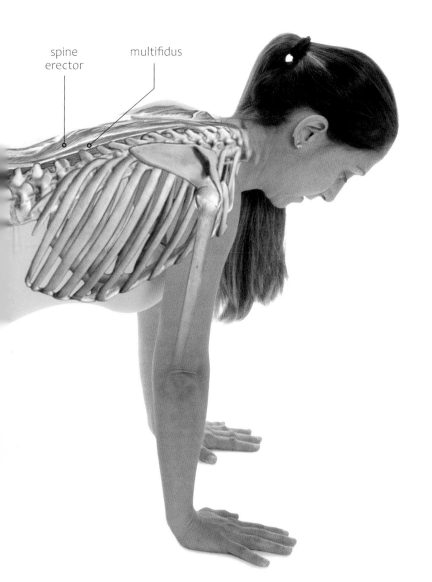

Squat Position

This position is good preparation for childbirth because it allows wide opening of the pelvis.

Stand with your feet and legs apart. Lower your hips to a squat position with your hands on the floor. Point your feet outward at an angle of about 45 degrees and bend your knees as much as you can in line with your ankles. Tilt your body forward. Place your forearms on the inside of your thighs with palms together. Face forward looking straight.

Slightly push your elbows outward with your knees to obtain a greater opening of the hips. Back stays straight and shoulders relaxed.

Remain in this position for several breaths. To release, place your hands on the floor and sit down.

- Leg and ankle reinforcement.

- The back muscles of the body are lengthened, relieving back pain.

- Opening of the pelvis and sacrum to promote descent and positioning of the baby.

- Connects pelvic floor and birth canal, helping with dilation between contractions.

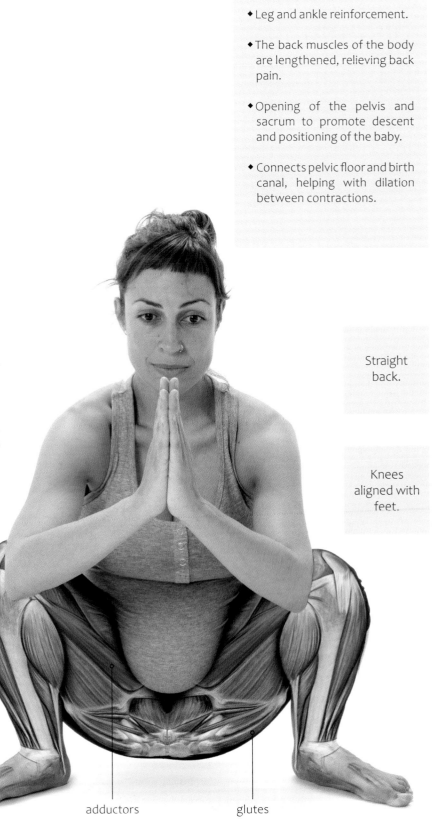

Straight back.

Knees aligned with feet.

Heels pressed against the floor.

adductors   glutes

⚠️

- For greater stability, perform the position by supporting your back against a wall.

- If you're not able to place the soles of your feet on the floor, place something under your heels.

- In case of contraindications, practice the modified position by sitting on a low bench or stool.

- Do not practice the modified position if you feel pain in your knees, prolapse of the cervix, threat of premature labor, placenta previa, fetus in breech position, varicose veins, and hemorrhoids.

Modification

Sitting on a bench or stool

Sit on a wide bench or low stool. Open your legs, knees in line with your feet. Back straight in neutral position and shoulders relaxed. Place your hands on your knees and hold the position breathing quietly.

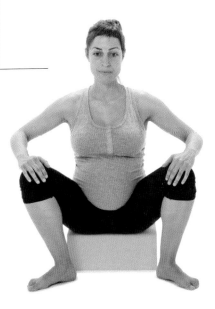

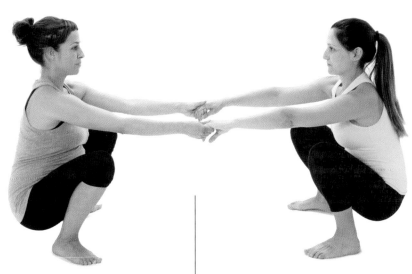

Variant

Couple squat position

Stand in front of your partner. Stretch out your arms and hold one another with your hands. Open your legs and start lowering your hips back and down until you are squatting in front of each other. Hold the position for a few breaths.

Tibial and Toe Extensor Stretching

This stretch relaxes the tibialis anterior and relieves pain in your legs and feet.

Kneel on the floor with your knees together. If the size of your belly makes it difficult, slightly spread your legs. Keep the outer edges of your thighs and hips aligned. Feet are in plantar flexion, knees to feet touching the floor.

Lower your hips and sit on your glutes touching your heels. Place your hands on your thighs or knees. Keep your chest expanded, back straight, and looking forward.

Stay in this position for a minute breathing quietly and release.

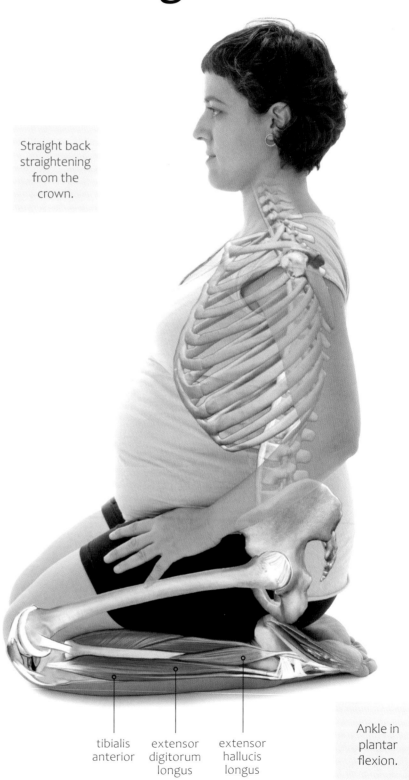

Straight back straightening from the crown.

tibialis anterior

extensor digitorum longus

extensor hallucis longus

Ankle in plantar flexion.

- Relieves tension in feet and strengthens front part of your feet.

- Prevents pain and swelling in legs.

- Reduces fatigue.

- If you have knee joint problems, perform with modifications.

- If you feel a lot of pressure on your knees or ankles, place a rolled blanket or bench between your glutes and heels as well as a small cushion under the front of your foot.

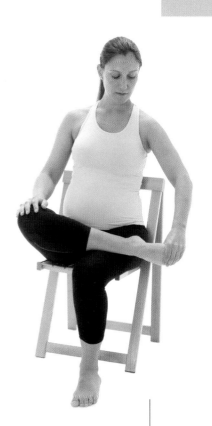

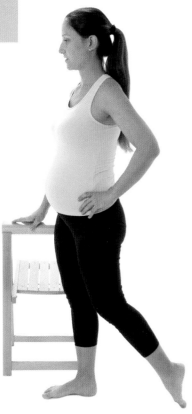

Variants

Toe flexion sitting in a chair

Sat in a chair with your back straight and the soles of your feet resting on the floor. Place your right leg on top of the left. With your right hand, grab your knee and with your left hand grab your toes. Stretch the front part of your foot and toes. Repeat with the opposite foot.

Static toe flexion on floor

Stand holding onto a chair to keep your balance. Bend your left leg at the knee and move it back. Support your toes on the floor. Press your foot lightly against the floor to stretch the entire front part of your foot and toe extenders. Hold this position for a few seconds and repeat with the opposite foot.

Pelvis Pivot with Lateral Hip Tilt

This dynamic stretch is a good exercise for pelvic waist mobility and preparation for childbirth.

Kneel on top of a blanket or mat, spread your legs at hip level and place your hands at the waist. Stretch from the crown upward and begin with chest (shallow) breathing. Leave space between the ribs and the abdomen.

Inhale and tilt your pelvis to the right, pulling your hip in the same direction. Hold this position for one breath. Return to the starting position, inhale again and tilt your pelvis to the left.

Repeat the two lateral movements slowly and continuously 6 to 10 times.

Face forward.

Shoulders relaxed.

quadratus lumborum

tensor fascia lata

gluteus medius

Avoid hyperlordosis of lower back.

Frontal plane movement.

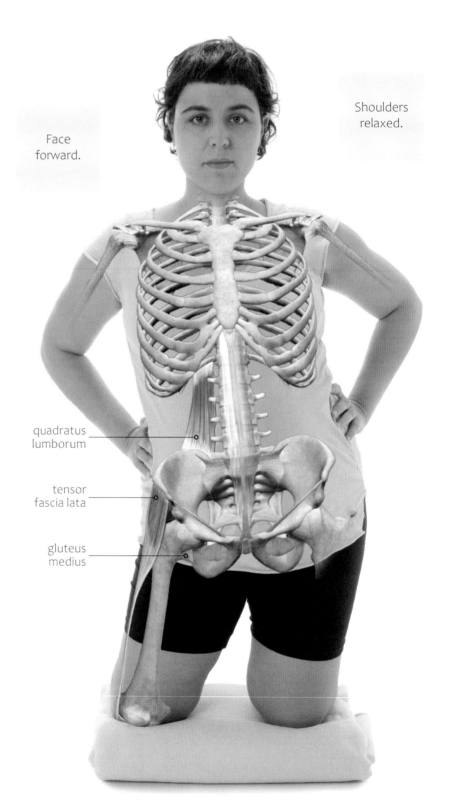

- Relieves hip pain.

- Relaxes the pelvis.

- Improves pelvic waist mobility.

Variants

Lateral tilt of the foot

Stand with legs apart and back straight. Hands rest on the hips. Bend the right leg slightly and swing your pelvis to the right. Slowly return to the starting position and tilt your pelvis to the left. Repeat the movement slowly and continuously.

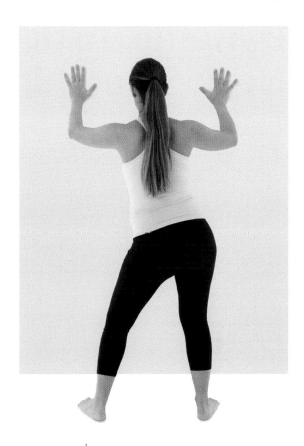

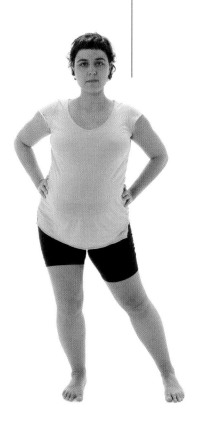

Lateral tilt against the wall

Stand in front of a wall with legs apart and knees slightly bent. Place both hands on the wall, with the palm of your hand open and arms parallel to the floor shoulder width apart. Perform the described lateral tilt first to one side and then to the other. Accompany the movement with slow, regular breathing.

Dynamic Articular Core Work: Neck Stretching

This stretch gives us flexibility in the dorsal and cervical area and allows us to work on our breathing.

Sit on a chair with your back straight and feet flat on the floor. Your legs can stay open. Place each hand on the corresponding knee with your palm facing down.

Inhale and extend your chest, bringing your body slightly forward. Keep your head aligned with your back, which is kept straight and scapula together (position one). Shoulders remain relaxed. The pelvis is slightly in anteversion.

When exhaling, the pelvis moves very slightly in retroversion. Bend the upper back by bending the torso. Lower your head and direct your chin toward your breastbone (position two). Separate your scapula. Shoulders remain relaxed.

Inhale and return to the starting position. Repeat the movement very slowly six to ten times.

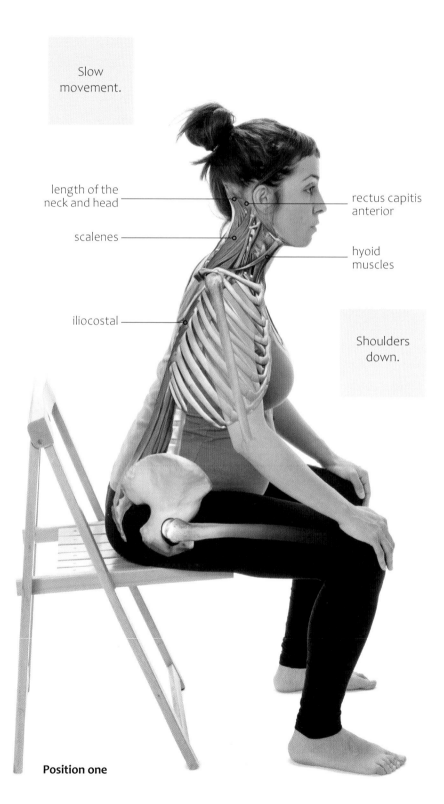

Slow movement.

length of the neck and head

rectus capitis anterior

scalenes

hyoid muscles

iliocostal

Shoulders down.

Sit on your glutes.

Position one

- Relieves and relaxes back muscles of the neck.

- Reduces tension and neck pain.

- Flexes the spine.

- Move slowly and in a controlled manner, otherwise you may feel dizzy.

- Cervical osteoarthritis problems.

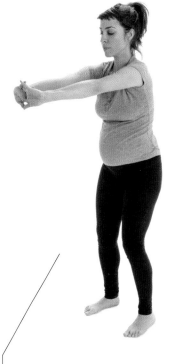

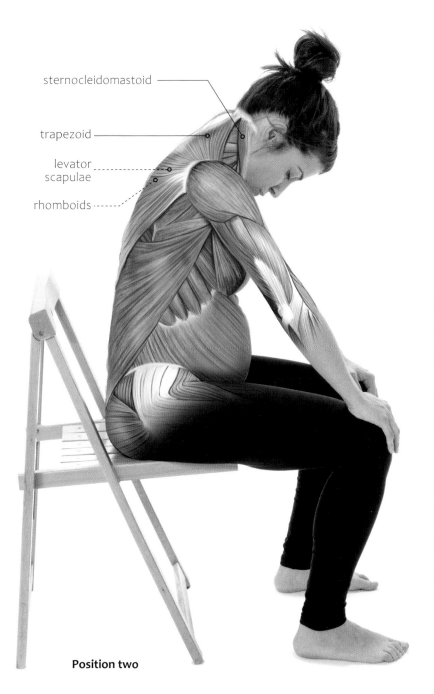

sternocleidomastoid

trapezoid

levator scapulae

rhomboids

Position two

Variants

Rhomboid stretch

Stand with your back straight, legs apart, and knees bent. Interlace the fingers of your hands and raise your arms a little below the height of your shoulders. Turn the palms of your hands and stretch your arms toward your forehead. Notice how your scapulae separate. Slightly lower your head. Hold the position for ten seconds and release.

Adductor Stretching

This stretch is a suitable position for practicing conscious breathing.

Sit on a block or low support with your back straight, head aligned, and your gaze forward. Bend your knees and place the soles of your feet together. Knees come down to the floor. The hands are placed above the knees. Shoulders remain relaxed.

Inhale and, with exhaling, slightly lift your body upward from the navel leaving space in the abdomen.

If you want to feel a greater stretch, sit in a lower seat. You can also lightly press on your knees with your hands toward the floor.

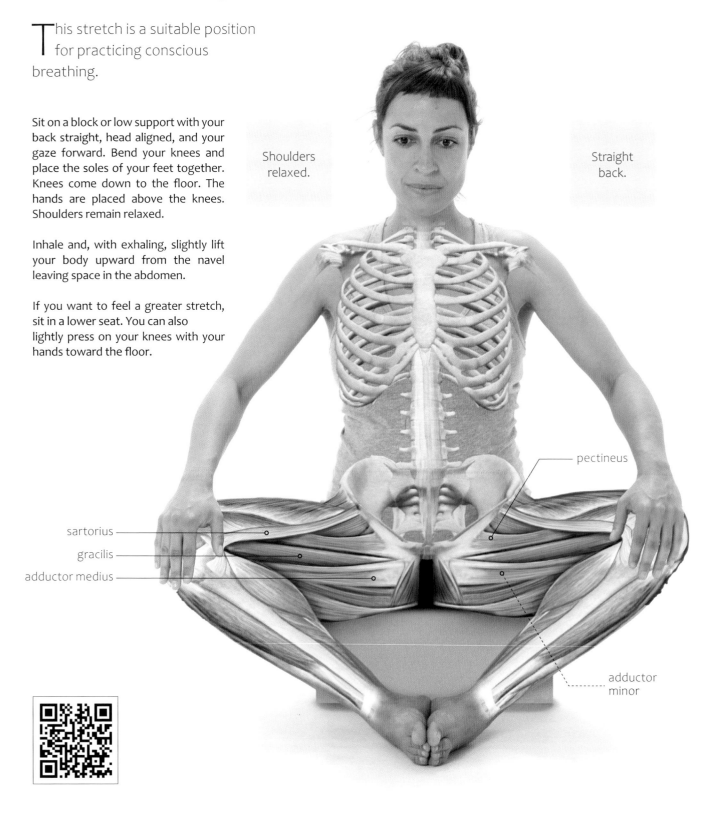

Shoulders relaxed.

Straight back.

pectineus

sartorius

gracilis

adductor medius

adductor minor

- Stretches your inner thighs and prepares you for delivery.

- Suitable position for practicing your breathing.

- Induces calm state and mental balance.

- To avoid back tension, lean against a wall.

- Meniscus knee problems.

- Pubic symphysis.

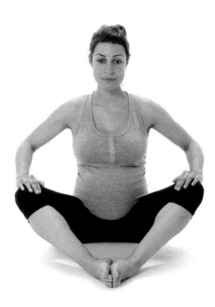

Stretching with legs apart

Sit on a bench, back straight. Spread your legs wide, knees and feet must remain aligned. Place the palms of your hands on the inside of your knees. Exhale and with your arms, slightly push your knees out. Repeat the movement three to six times.

Variants

Dynamic stretch

As in the initial exercise, sit on a bench with the soles of your feet together. Back straight. Inhale, and while exhaling, gently press your knees toward the floor with your hands to intensify the stretch. Hold for a few seconds and relax. Repeat the stretch three to six times.

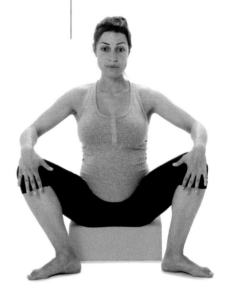

Quadruped Pelvic Circles

This is a joint mobility exercise. It helps prepare for the time of delivery by releasing the pelvis and sacrum, giving them freedom of movement.

Go on all fours on top of a folded blanket. Spread your legs so you have a wide base for support. Carry the weight of your body on your knees. Hands are placed on the floor with palms open and active.

Make circular movements with the hips. The movement must be fluid and slow and without reaching maximum joint amplitude. Be aware of your pelvic movements. You can also make circular, figure-eight movements.

Repeat the movements on one side 6 to 10 times and then make circles toward the opposite side.

Do not reach maximum joint amplitude.

gluteus medius

gluteus minimus

gluteus maximus

quadratus lumborum

abdominal obliques

rectus abdominis

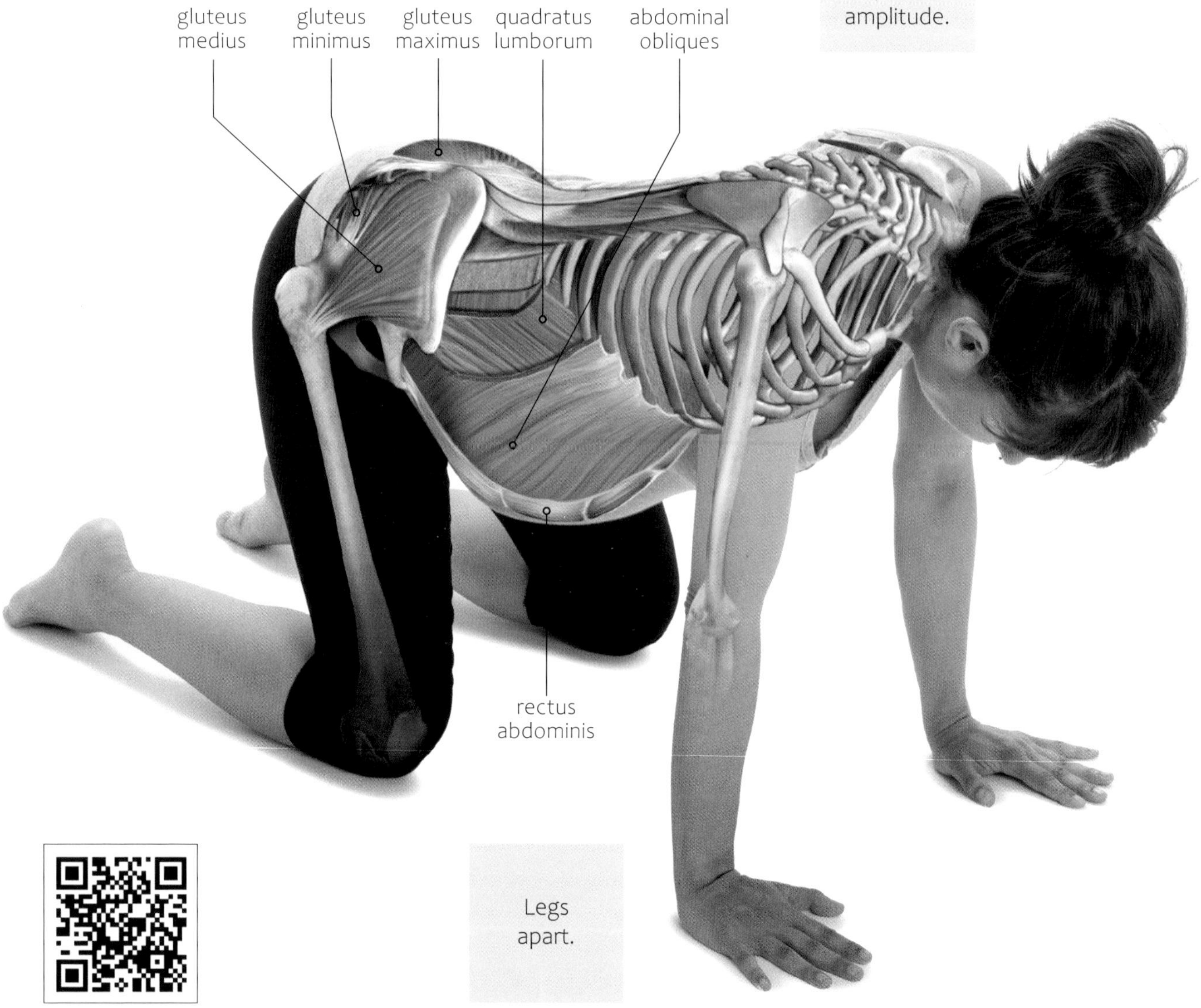

Legs apart.

- Prepares for delivery.

- Provides pelvic mobility.

- Relaxes the pelvis, lumbar, and sacrum.

- If you have wrist problems, perform the exercise by keeping your body on pillows or a large ball.

Variants

Pelvic circles with wall support

Stand facing a wall with your hands open. Spread your legs and notice how your feet rest on the floor. Slowly make circles with your hips to one side and then the other. You can raise one leg by placing a small cushion under one foot and do asymmetrical circles.

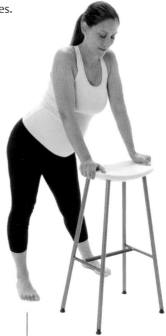

Pelvic circles using a bench

Support yourself on a bench, spread your legs apart and feel your feet against the floor. You can make various movements with your hips, for example, drawing small circles, making big circles, keeping more weight on one leg, carrying the weight of one leg toward the other, etc. You can also perform circles with one leg rotating inward or out. All these movements prepare the pelvis, making childbirth easier.

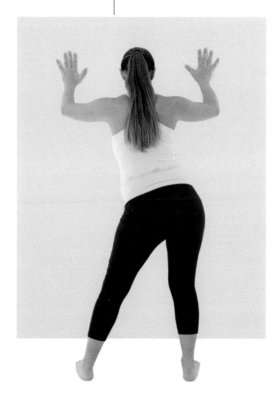

Postpartum Stretching

After delivery, it is necessary to help the body recover. Resting, Kegel exercises, and hypopressive abdominal work will initially be helpful. It is not advisable to start exercising until six weeks after delivery and ten weeks in the case of a cesarean section. Practice exercising again gradually with no rush to regain your physique.

In this chapter, we will explain exercises aimed at recovering your abdomen and pelvic floor as these are the areas that have been altered the most. Classic ab work is completely contraindicated since this increases intra-abdominal pressure, contributing to distension and placing pressure on the perineum.

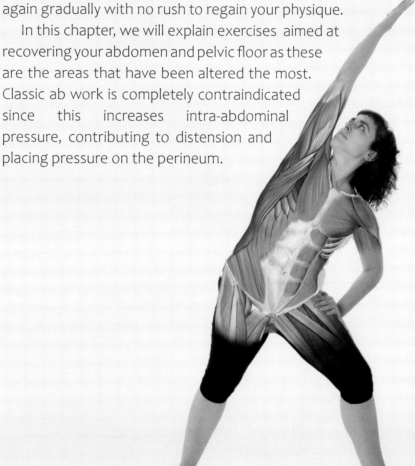

Hypopressive Ab and Pelvic Floor Exercises

Hypopressive exercises favor the abdomen tone by lowering abdominal pressure.

Lie in supine position with legs bent and heels on the floor. Aligned spine, neutral pelvis. Stretch starting from the crown of your head.

Raise your arms to shoulder height, in internal rotation. The palms of your hands face up with the tips of your fingers touching each other. Elbows flex slightly. Push up with your shoulder blades.

Breathe in and out gently through your mouth, activating your pelvic floor and transverse abdominals by bringing your navel toward the spine and upward as if you were trying to close a zipper from the pelvis.

Breathe in and out again, gently releasing all the air until the lungs are completely emptied. While exhaling, push your arms up, opening the ribs ready for costal breathing.

Pull the navel to the floor and up. Hold for a few seconds and slowly release the movement while slowly inhaling.

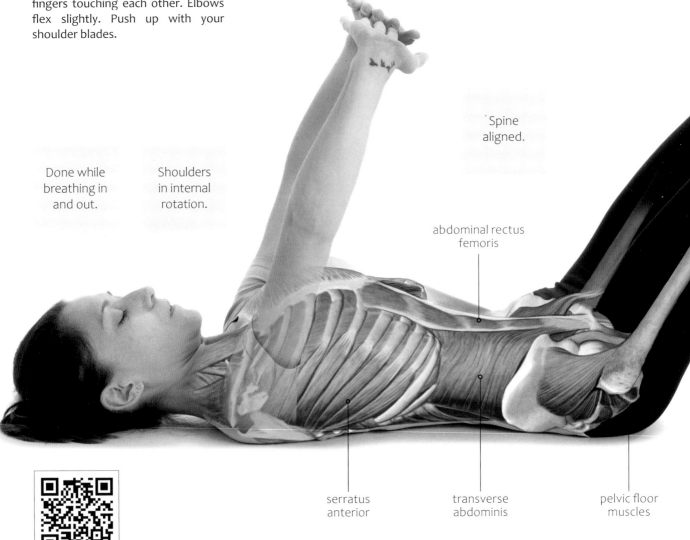

Done while breathing in and out.

Shoulders in internal rotation.

Spine aligned.

abdominal rectus femoris

serratus anterior

transverse abdominis

pelvic floor muscles

- Posture correction and prevents back pain.

- Along with pelvic floor exercises, reduces the risk of urinary incontinence, hernias, and prolapse.

- These tone up abdominal muscles recovering their functionality.

- Treatment of diastasis recti.

- Improvement of intestinal movements.

- Pregnancy, hypertension, heart disease, and obstructive respiratory dysfunction.

Variants

Stand up and step forward with one leg in front of the other. Knees are slightly bent. Arms are at shoulder level, elbows bent, and palms facing forward with fingertips. Your shoulders remain down and your scapula are separated. Stretch your spine from the crown upward. Slightly move your weight forward. Breathe in through your nose and let the air out through your mouth. Activate the pelvic floor and the abdominal waist as if it were a zipper that closes from the pelvis to the sternum. Inhale again and deeply release the air. Close your throat and do costal breathing by opening the ribs and raising the navel up and back while raising your arms forward. Hold for three seconds and let go of the movement by slowly inhaling. Repeat the exercise up to seven times.

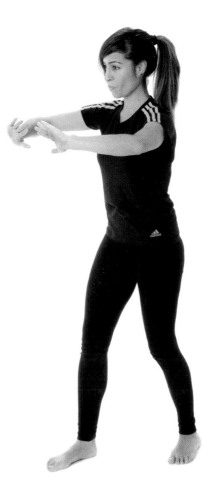
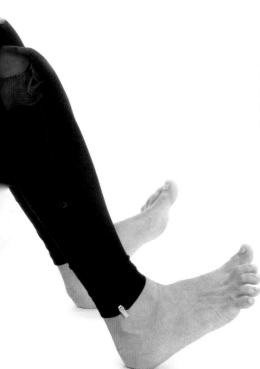

Back Extension: The Sphinx

These stretches strengthen the spine extensors and help develop mobility in the upper back.

Lie in prone position with a neutral spine. Rest your forehead on a mat. Spread your legs apart at hip level and arms bent at the side of your body.

Inhale and, when exhaling, raise your head, neck, and chest with the strength of your back.

Contract your glutes and move them as if you wanted to push them toward your heels. Your navel should be pulled upward and inward. Elbows are flexed and positioned at shoulder level. Forearm and palms of your hands are in contact with the floor.

Raise your lower ribs by pressing down with your forearms. The pelvis remains in contact with the ground. Open your shoulders and pull your shoulder blades down to expand the chest.

Hold this position and breathe calmly. Be conscious of how your chest expands.

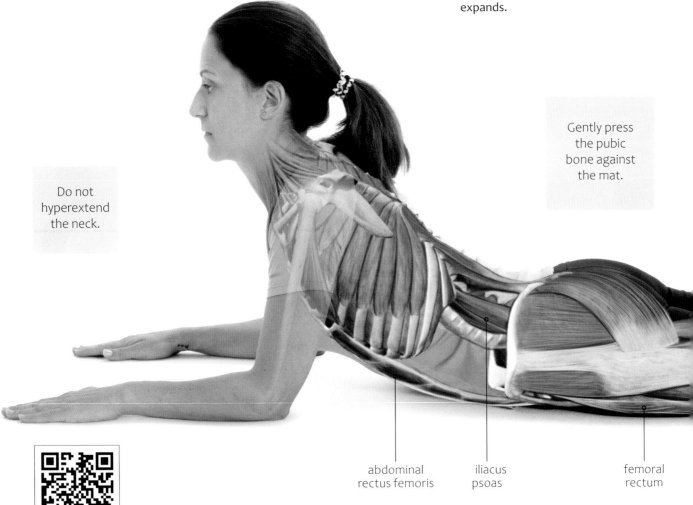

Do not hyperextend the neck.

Gently press the pubic bone against the mat.

abdominal rectus femoris

iliacus psoas

femoral rectum

- Strengthens spine extensors.

- Improves posture and expands the chest.

⚠

- Problems in the lumbar spine (sciatica, hernias).

- Abdominal hernias.

Variants

Simple variant with hands on shoulders

In prone position, pelvis in neutral position, arms crossed and head supported. Inhale and exhale and lift your head and chest off the floor. Keep your lower ribs in contact with the ground. The spine stretches and the chest opens. Use your arms as support to maintain your position. Hold for a few breaths and, as you exhale, slowly release. Repeat 6 to 10 times.

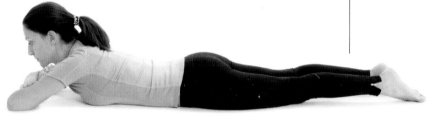

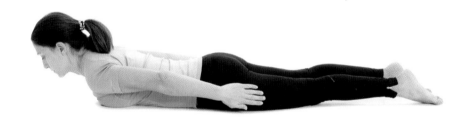

Prone spine extension

In prone position, place your legs together and feet in dorsal flexion. Support your forehead on the mat and stretch your arms along the body. The spine and pelvis are in a neutral position. Inhale and exhale, stretch your arms and, with using your back muscles, raise your head, neck, and chest. The lower ribs should remain glued to the mat. The legs are also stretched. The palms of your hands should face your body, and your feet remain in contact with the mat. Face downward. Hold this position for two breaths and release when you exhale. Repeat 6 to 10 times.

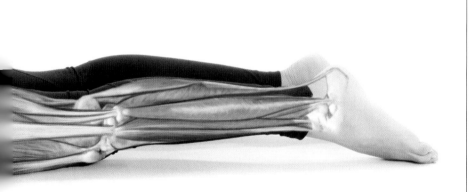

Core Anterior Flexion and Hamstring Stretching

This posture stretches the back of the legs and tones the back muscles.

Sit on a blanket with legs bent close to your body. Your abdomen and thighs are touching. Stretch your back and grab your toes with your hands. Slowly slide your legs forward.

Stretch your legs a little further and elongate the spine. Relax your head and shoulders. If you cannot reach your feet with your hands when extending your legs, they can rest on your legs.

Hold the position for a few minutes by breathing quietly.

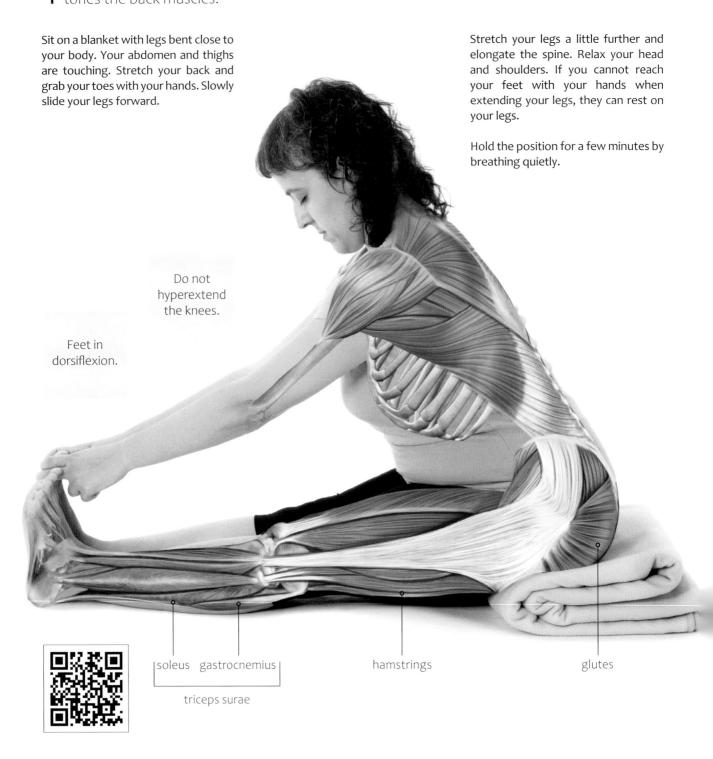

Do not hyperextend the knees.

Feet in dorsiflexion.

soleus   gastrocnemius

triceps surae

hamstrings

glutes

- Stretches the posterior part of your legs.

- Stimulates abdominal organs.

- Relaxes the nervous system.

⚠

- If you have problems in your spine, such as hernias disc, sciatica, or lumbago, perform the variant in supine position.

- In case of back stiffness or shortening of the hamstrings, you can place a band to hold the position and stretch the back.

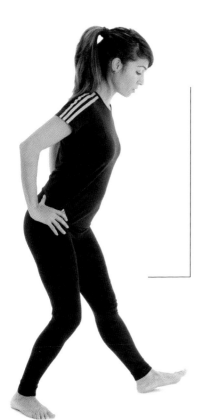

Variants

Standing hamstring stretch

Take a step forward with your left leg. Place your hands on your waist. Bend and move the weight to your right leg. The left leg remains straight and rests on the heel. With a straight back, bend your body forward until you feel the stretch. Take a few breaths and repeat on the opposite side.

Supine hamstring stretch

Lie in a supine position with your legs flexed and the soles of your feet resting on the floor. Bring one leg toward your body and with the help of a band placed on the metatarsals of your foot, vertically extend your leg, feeling the stretch in your hamstrings.

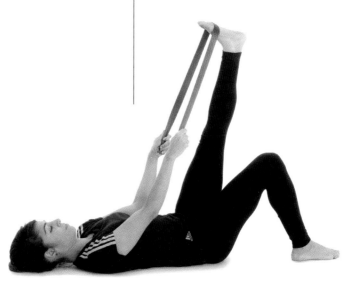

Abdominal Muscle Activation

The abdominal muscles are worked by initiating movement with activation of the transversus abdominis, which is the deepest musculature to continue activating the rectus abdominis and oblique muscles.

In a supine position with your knees bent, legs bent at a straight angle with thighs, and soles of feet resting on the floor at hip level. Pelvis in neutral position, stretch your spine by keeping your back elongated.

Inhale and exhale by contracting the perineum. Activate the transverse abdominis and lift your right leg up until your thigh is perpendicular to the floor and knee is aligned with your hip.

Hold this position for a few breaths and lower your leg slowly. Your pelvis remains stable without bending your lumbar spine.

Do this exercise six times and repeat with the opposite leg.

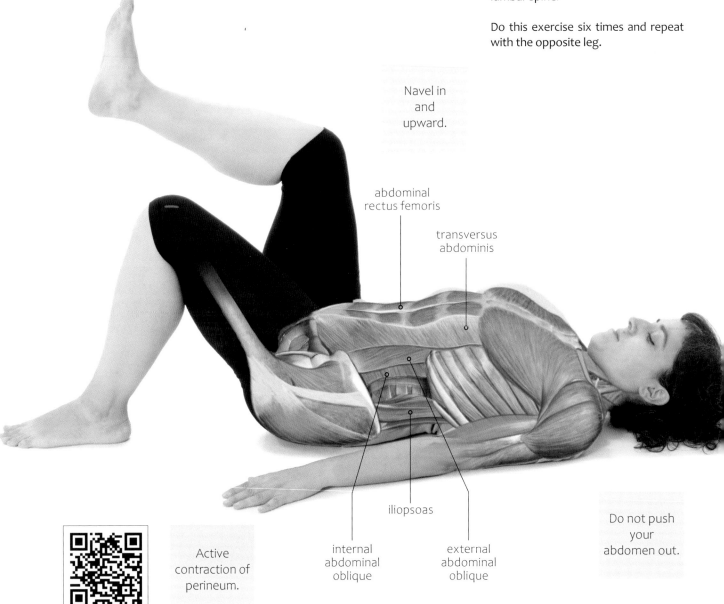

Navel in and upward.

abdominal rectus femoris

transversus abdominis

Active contraction of perineum.

iliopsoas

internal abdominal oblique

external abdominal oblique

Do not push your abdomen out.

◉

• Accelerates recovery from diastasis recti.

• Stabilizes the lower back and pelvis.

• If activated with pelvic floor, this tones the latter.

⚠

• It is very important to control your lumbar area by pushing your navel in and up to keep the transversus abdominis active. Keep your pelvis stable when raising or lowering your leg.

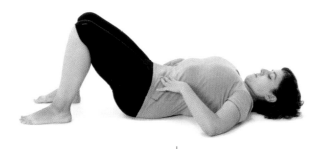

Variants

Activation of transversus abdominis

Lie in a supine position with your legs bent and the soles of your feet on the floor. The pelvis is in neutral position. Gently exhale and activate your transversus abdominis by gently pushing your navel in and up. Imagine you are zipping up a tight-fitting pair of pants. Hold the position for a few seconds, inhale, and release. Repeat the movement ten times.

To ensure you are activating the transversus abdominis, place your fingers above your iliac crests.

Transversus abdominis and major and minor oblique exercises

Start from the same position as before. Place the sole of your right foot on your left knee. Raise your right arm and support your forearm on the right knee. Activate your transversus abdominis and push your arm toward your knee and your knee toward your arm. Relax and repeat 6 to 10 times. Repeat on the other side.

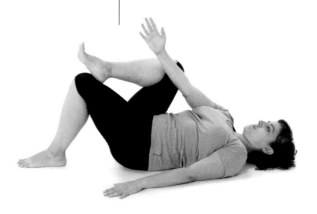

Forearm Plank

The plank strengthens the muscles of the core by improving resistance and toning your abdomen.

Lie on all fours with arms and knees apart at hip level. Bend your arms by placing your forearms and elbows slightly away from your shoulders and touching the ground. Put the palms of your hands together and interlace your fingers. Your arms should be perpendicular to the ground.

Activate your pelvic floor and transversus abdominis by moving your navel up and back. Stretch one leg first and then the other, resting your toes on the floor.

Your back should remain straight and the spine elongated, stretching from the crown and pushing with your heels in the opposite direction. Weight is distributed between your forearms and toes. Do not bend your lumbar spine. Keep your pelvis in neutral position. Hold the position by breathing through your ribs.

Do for five seconds and rest. Repeat three times. You can increase the time as you become stronger. Ideally you should be able to hold the position for at least 20 seconds.

Pelvis in neutral position and aligned with your core and legs.

abdominal obliques

iliopsaas

transversus abdominis

serratus anterior

abdominal rectus femoris

Arms perpendicular to the ground.

Do not hold your breath.

- Strengthens spine, hips. and arms.

- Tones the abdomen.

- Do not push out your abdomen. To do this, you must activate the transversus abdominis.

- Air is carried to the ribs when inhaling. Do not hold hold your breath.

- It is not recommended for people with lumbar problems.

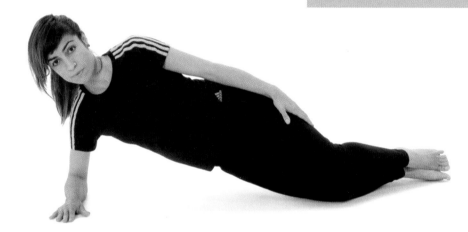

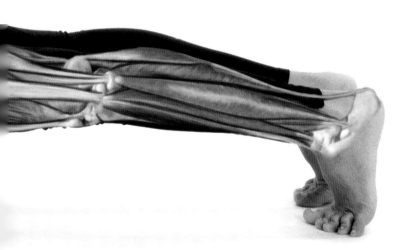

Variants

Side plank

In a lateral position, lean against your forearm on the floor. Knees should stay bent and in contact with the floor. Stretch your spine so it stays in neutral position. Contract the transversus abdominis, push your hips up and lift your pelvis and core together as you exhale. Hold for five seconds, breathing through your ribs and lowering yourself down.

Leg and Arm Elevation

The isometric work of the rectus abdominis keeps these at a constant length, thus avoiding intervertebral disc compression and pressure in the perineum.

In a supine position, place your legs hip width apart and bent at the knees. Place the soles of your feet on the ground. You can stabilize your pelvis by placing a small blanket under your lumbar spine.

Inhale through the ribs, exhale and activate the perineum, transversus abdominis and elevate both bent legs and arms.

Hold for a few breaths. Exhale and slowly lower your legs and arms toward the floor.

This position can be repeated three times. Maintenance time will increase as you get stronger.

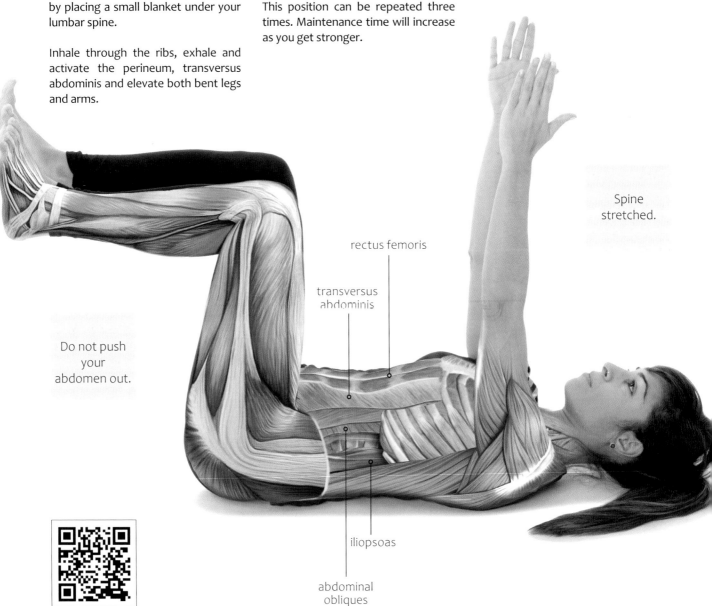

Spine stretched.

rectus femoris

transversus abdominis

Do not push your abdomen out.

iliopsoas

abdominal obliques

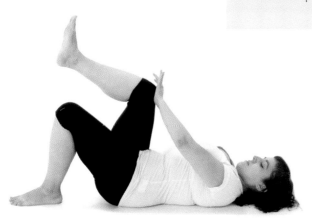

- Strengthens abdominal muscles.

- Tones the quadriceps.

- Exercises involving shortening of the rectus abdominis are not advisable and are contraindicated if there is diastasis of the abdomen.

- In case of dynamic abdominal exercises, maintain an opening of the ribs through rib or costal breathing. Do not block the glottis nor hold your breath while doing the exercise to avoid pressure on the perineum.

Variants

Isometric oblique and rectus abdominis contraction

Lie in a supine position with legs bent and soles of feet on the ground. Raise your left leg, bent by the knee, bringing it toward your body until your thigh is perpendicular to the ground.

Grab the knee of your left leg with your right hand. Inhale, exhale, and activate the transversus abdominis and perineum. While breathing, push your hand against your knee to bring down the leg that remains in the same position. Inhale and relax. Repeat the process 6 to 10 times and change arm and leg.

Rectus abdominis contraction with head elevation

When performing dynamic ab work, you must be aware of your perineum, contracting so that it does not put pressure on the abdomen. Lay in a supine position with knees bent and soles of feet resting on the ground separated at hip level. Tilt your pelvis. Place your hands with the tips of your fingers touching your cervical spine.

Inhale from your rib cage. Exhale and contract the perineum, activate your transversus abdominis and, while keeping your rib cage open, slightly raise your head and shoulders. Exhale through your mouth. Inhale and lay back down on the ground. Keep your lower back against the floor throughout the whole exercise. Do not block the glottis during the exercise. Repeat 6 to 10 times.

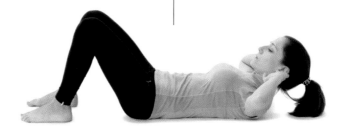

Leg and Arm Elevation 123

Arm, Neck, and Shoulder Stretching

These stretches lighten forearms, neck, and shoulder pain due to overload that usually appears in these areas during the postpartum period.

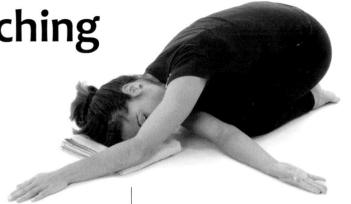

Arm flexor stretching

On all fours, rotate your arms out so that the fingers of your hands are facing toward your knees with thumbs facing out. Your arms remain extended. To intensify the stretch, gently move your body back. Hold the stretch for a few breaths and release. Repeat three times.

Trapezoid stretching. Assisted lateral flexing

On your knees, place your right arm behind your back and your left hand at the top of your head. Gently, tilt the neck to the left with your hand, directing your ear toward your shoulder. Hold the stretch for a few seconds and bring your head back to the center. Do not force the stretch. Repeat on the opposite side.

Middle trapezoid stretch

Sit on your knees over your heels and stretch your arms by sliding your hands forward. Pass your right arm under your body touching the floor with your palms facing upward, and stretch your arm away from your shoulder. Rotate your body and head toward the left. If necessary, place a cushion under your head.

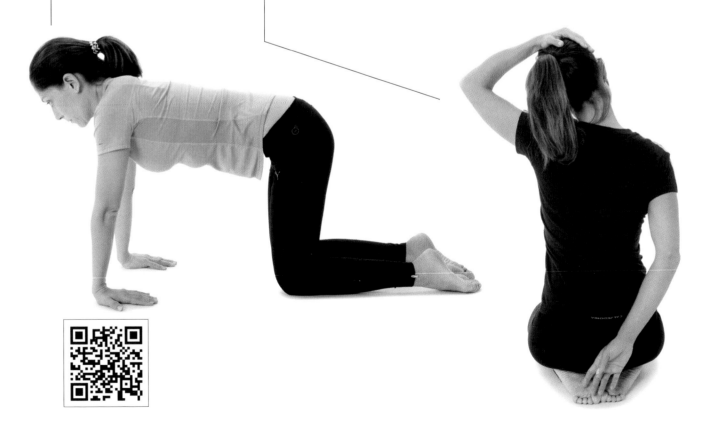

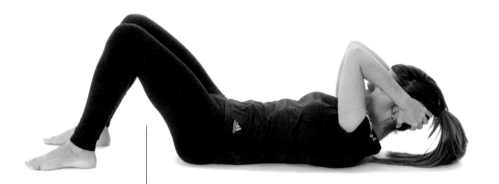

Upper and middle trapezoid stretch

Stretch your legs with the soles of the feet touching each other. Place the palm of one hand on the back of the opposite hand and pull forward. Follow the movement with your head.

Neck stretching (suboccipital, semispinalis, splenius)

In a supine position, flex your legs at hip level and place the soles of your feet on the floor. Tilt your pelvis so that you feel your lumbar spine touching the ground. Relax the pelvis. Take your head with your hands. Your thumbs can be placed at the base of your skull. Inhale, exhale, and raise your head with your hands gently bringing it forward with your chin pointing toward your chest, lengthening the cervical part. Your elbows should be near each other. Tilt your pelvis so that your lumbar spine is back against the floor. Pushing downward with your head. Hold one full breath and release.
Repeat three times.

Shoulder blade mobilization

In a supine position, bend your legs and place the soles of your feet on the floor. Your pelvis should be in a neutral position. Raise your arms vertically, parallel to shoulder height and with your palms facing each other. Inhale and raise both arms at the same time toward the sky. While exhaling, gently lower them. Keep your pelvis static and neck relaxed at all times. Repeat about 10 times.

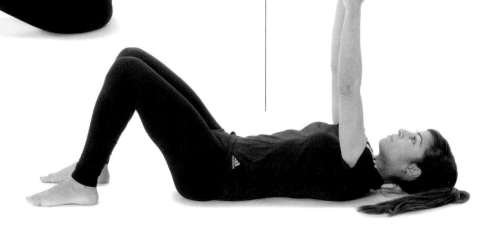

Rectus Abdominis Stretching

These stretches allow us to become aware of our deep breathing, opening up the ribs and inducing a state of calm.

- ◆ Stretches the front of the body.
- ◆ Improves shoulder mobility.
- ◆ Tones abdominal organs and expands the chest.

In a supine position, bend your legs and place the soles of your feet on the floor. Arms are positioned at the side of the body. Place a folded blanket under your lumbar area. Bring hands together and pull arms up in front of your chest.

Inhale and move your arms back while your legs stretch toward the floor. Hold a few breaths noticing the opening of your rib cage with each inhalation.

You can lengthen the stretch a little by taking your hands away from your head and feet in the opposite direction (both dorsal flexion and plantar flexion) as long as you don't feel tension.

Breathe out and return slowly to the starting position. Repeat several times. Release and relax.

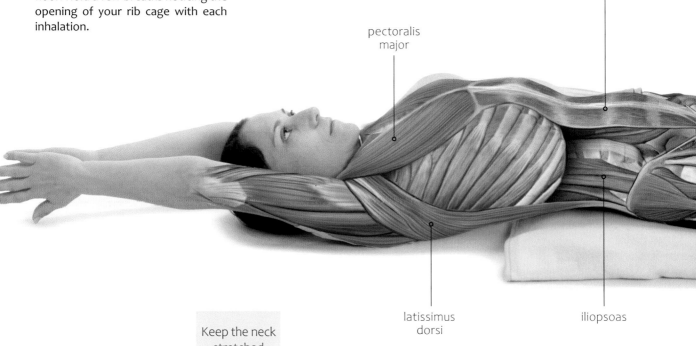

abdominal
rectus femoris

pectoralis
major

latissimus
dorsi

iliopsoas

Keep the neck
stretched
without
tension.

Maintains
curvature
of lumbar
spine.

⚠️

- If you feel shoulder discomfort, bend your arms at the elbows, stretch gently and don't raise the arms as high.

- If you feel lower back discomfort, keep your legs bent.

- The arms should find a place to hold onto. You can use a pillow if they do not touch the floor.

- In case of cesarean section, exercise when the wound is completely healed.

- The thickness of the blanket increases the stretch. Practice with caution.

Variants

Lateral position stretch

Lie in a lateral position with your right leg folded and your left arm extended up and back. Twist your whole body toward your left side so that this side is laying on the mat. Both legs are extended. Hold for a moment, inhale, and bring your right arm upward, bringing the palms of your hands together. Your upper arm and leg stretch slowly, growing, and creating space. Hold this position for a few breaths and release. Then, repeat on the opposite side.

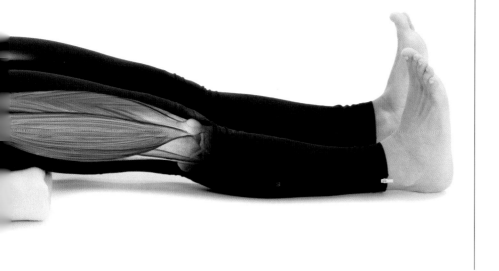

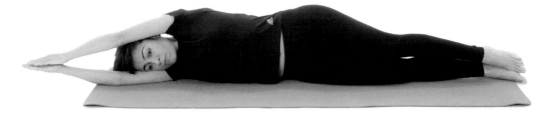

Abdominal Oblique Stretching

These stretches increase your spine flexibility and awareness of your breathing.

Stand up, legs apart, and turn your right foot out. Spread your weight between both legs. The pelvis is in neutral position. Your bent leg is aligned with your foot, and your knee should not exceed ankle height. Place your right hand on the thigh of the bent leg so that the stretched muscles are not activated.

Inhale through your ribs and raise your left arm upward above your head, accompanying a lateral flexion of the core. If you are flexible enough, place your right forearm on your thigh. Do not bend your body forward. The legs, core, hips, and arms must be in the same plane.

Hold the stretch for a few breaths and relax. Repeat on the opposite side.

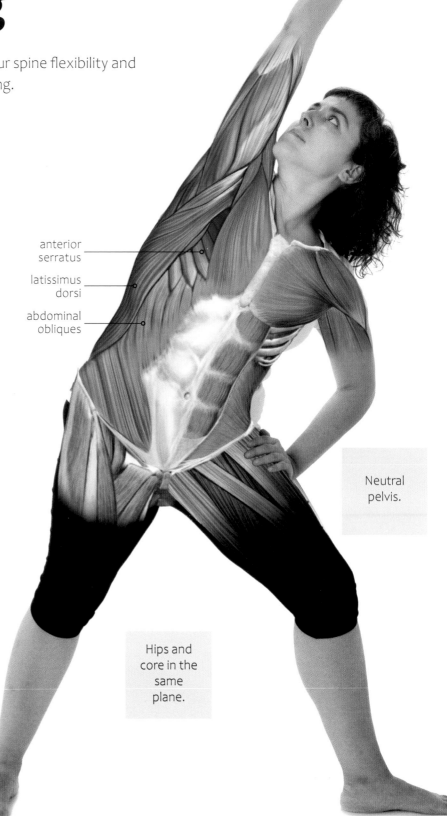

anterior serratus

latissimus dorsi

abdominal obliques

Neutral pelvis.

Hips and core in the same plane.

- Increases flexibility of the spine.

- Stimulates breathing and circulation.

- Improves body posture.

- In the event of lumbar spine injuries, stretch with caution.

Variants

Minor oblique stretching with crossed legs

Stand with your legs slightly bent. Pass the weight to your right leg, which bends slightly more at the knee. Take a step back with your left leg and cross behind your right leg. Distribute your weight between the legs. Rest your right hand on your right hip while the left arm rises above your head and accompanies the lateral flexion. Hold for a few breaths. Release and repeat on the opposite side.

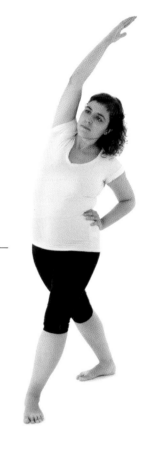

Lateral chain stretch in supine position

Lie in a supine position, back and pelvis in a neutral position. Bend your left leg by placing your foot on the floor and moving it away from your body to the left. Bring your straight right leg to the left leg, while raising your right arm and stretching toward your head. Try to stretch your entire side by slightly arching your body. Hold for a few breaths and slowly release. Repeat on the opposite side.

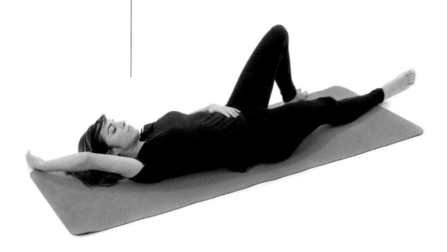

Breathing and Relaxation

Conscious breathing is a source of well-being and our great ally in both pregnancy and childbirth. Inhaling and exhaling more slowly and deeply provides physical and psychological benefits.

This final chapter explains how to breathe consciously as well as other breathing techniques that, in addition to improving oxygenation and relaxation, are effective at the time of delivery. We complete the chapter by showing you how to relax and perform visualizations to allow the body and mind to rest.

Breathing and Pregnancy

Throughout our pregnancy, we experience various emotions that will influence our mood and physiological processes. Conscious breathing is our great ally during pregnancy, at time of delivery, and in the upbringing of the baby.

Emotions and Breathing

During pregnancy, women face profound transformation in a short space of time. Throughout this period, all kinds of intense emotions can be experienced that have a direct impact on our breathing. When we experience intense emotion, fear, stress, or pain, our breathing becomes more superficial, faster, and shorter. However, in moments where we are more relaxed or rested, breathing becomes more leisurely, rhythmic, and slow.

The objective is to learn how to breathe slowly and deeply to calm your nervous system so you can face any situation calmly that arises during pregnancy.

Conscious Breathing and Pregnancy

To practice breathing exercises, find a posture where you feel comfortable and stable. Breathing will be done primarily through the nose, but in some cases, it can also be done through the mouth. Before beginning any modifications to your breathing, it is necessary to be aware of your natural breathing.

Awareness of Natural Breathing
Sit comfortably with your back straight and eyes closed. Relax your arms, shoulders, and face. Pay close attention to your breathing without attempting to make any changes to it. Observe as the air enters and leaves through your nostrils, notice its temperature, sound, intensity, and rhythm.

To practice breathing exercises, find a posture where you feel comfortable and stable, such as:
1. *Abdominal breathing. Arms and shoulders stay relaxed.*
2. *Thoracic-costal breathing.*
3. *Clavicle breathing.*

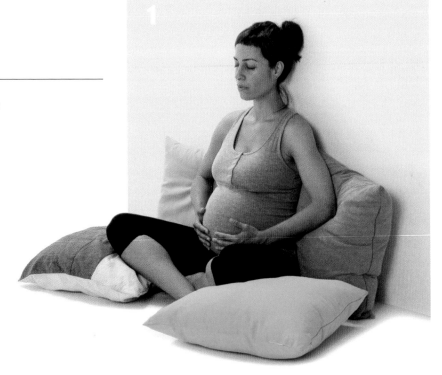

1. Abdominal breathing

Place your hands on your abdomen. Inhale and carry the air into the lower part of your lungs and watch how your abdomen rises as you breathe in and falls as you breathe out. Lengthen your exhale and feel that, at the same time, you are relaxing your body and thoughts.

2. Thoracic-costal breathing

Place both hands at rib height, and while inhaling, try to expand your chest to the sides and up.

3. Clavicle breathing

Very shallow breaths can be felt by placing your hands on top of the clavicles.

- Increases perception and concentration.

- Oxygenates the body by eliminating fatigue.

- Relaxes the nervous system promoting a calm state.

- Increases stress resistance.

- Increases vitality and energy.

- It connects you with your baby.

- It allows good oxygenation for the baby.

- Prepares you for delivery.

⚠

- Breathing **should never be forced** as it may induce hyperventilation. In every breath, respect your natural rhythm. The objective is to breath in a deeper, rhythmic, and slower way.

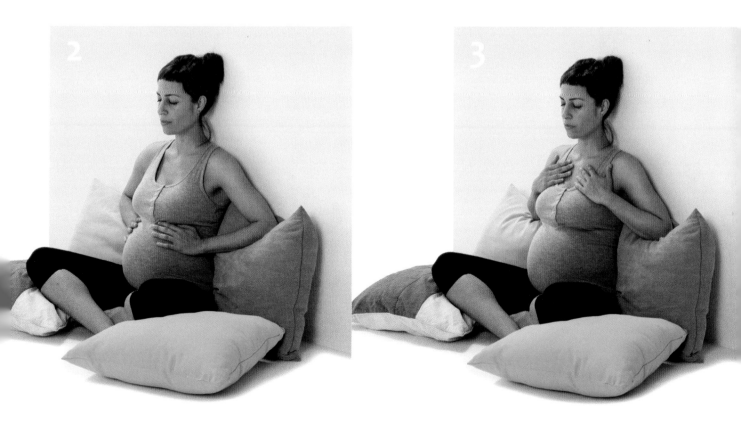

Breathing Practice

As you have seen, there is a connection between the way we breathe and our physical and emotional state. Through simple respiratory practices, we can influence our mood and even our perception of pain. The continued practice of deep breathing will allow you to calm your mind and help you at the time of delivery.

Respiratory Rate and Rhythm

The rate is the number of breaths that we take at a given time. Normally, in a healthy adult, the rate is 12 to 20 breaths per minute. In the case of a pregnant woman, the respiratory rate is modified slightly, usually by one to two breaths per minute (15%).

Breathing rhythm is the regularity of time we spend on inhaling and exhaling, as well as whether there is a small moment between them when we aren't breathing. The practices of conscious breathing allow us to voluntarily modify this rhythm for different purposes. Balanced breathing is when the duration of inhaling and exhaling are equal (1:1); relaxed breathing is when exhaling is slower and longer than inhaling (1:2).

Full Breathing

To practice full breathing, place one hand on your abdomen and the other on your chest.

At first you will observe your natural breathing and, little by little, you will perform breathing that will affect the three respiratory zones. To do this, begin inhaling by bringing the air toward your abdominal area and, from there, spread it gently to the thoracic-costal and clavicle areas. When exhaling, air is expelled from the abdominal area first. If we voluntarily lengthen our exhaling, we will calm the mind and relax the nervous system.

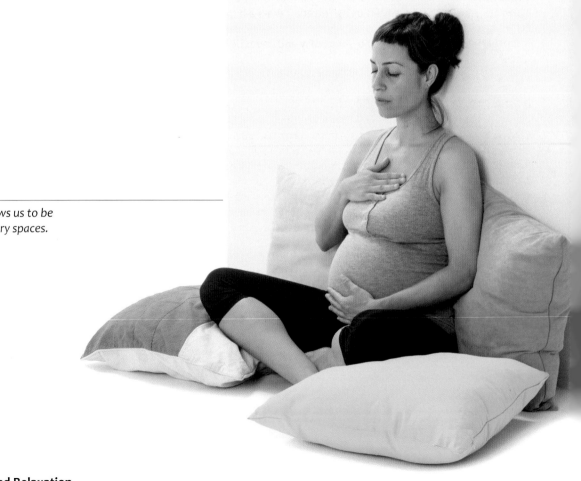

Full breathing allows us to be aware of respiratory spaces.

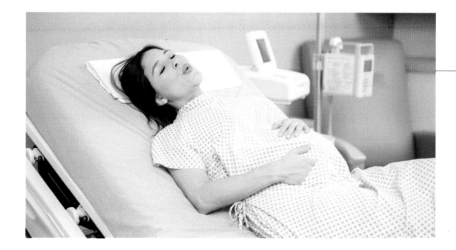

Contractions can be visualized as waves coming in and out.

Ujjayi Breathing

This is a breathing method that produces a great calm and increases internalization. You can practice it by partially closing the glottis when breathing so that the air coming in and out is slowed down. It can also be performed only when exhaling. To do this, take chest breaths, and when exhaling, partially close the glottis and draw the air slowly through the nose, observing the sound it makes. Exhalation should last longer than inhalation.

A modification could be to blow the air out of your mouth producing a long sound using letters: "A-a-a-a-h", "U-u-u-u-u-h."

Precautions: inhalation must flow naturally and never be forced.

Breathing During Labor

Breathing is our great ally in the labor process. Each woman must find her own way of breathing, adapting it to the needs of the moment. If conscious breaths have been practiced during pregnancy, these will be present and arise spontaneously. Here are some breathing techniques that may be useful in synchronizing with your uterus, coping with pain, and helping yourself and your baby through the process.

During childbirth we can distinguish a dilation phase, a transition phase, and an expulsion phase. In the first phase, contractions will be spaced apart. Little by little they become more frequent until they become very intense in the expulsion phase. We will distinguish three types of breathing according to the phases.

In the **dilation phase**, breathing must be natural between contractions. During a contraction, deep breaths in can be performed through the mouth, emitting a sound as in Ujjayi breathing or in a more acoustic manner by pronouncing letters or consonants.

As labor progresses, we enter a **transition phase** where contractions are more frequent and breathing becomes faster. At the peak of the contractions, and if these are very strong, you can breathe by gasping three to four times (shortness of breath) through the mouth or nose and exhaling through the mouth in a long, deep, and loud manner. Complete this respiratory pattern before the contraction ends.

Finally, in the **expulsion phase**, take a breath in and follow the push by exhaling intensely, letting out the air through your mouth as if you were whistling.

Postpartum Breathing

You can take calming breaths such as the *Ujjayi* breaths and full breathing during postpartum. You can also practice with your baby so that their breathing is synchronized with yours. If we maintain calm and deep breathing, we will transmit tranquility and confidence to the newborn.

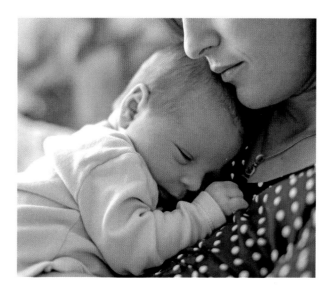

Relaxation and Visualization

Relaxation practices combined with visualization techniques are excellent tools for promoting a calm physical and mental state. They improve the well-being of the pregnant woman and her baby.

Relaxation

Relaxation gives us the opportunity to let go of the body and clearly perceive our inner state. It also allows us to recover energy in a short time. It is advisable, after practicing stretches, to relax for about 10 to 15 minutes. This enables a moment of rest and calm.

At the time of delivery and during the whole process, it is great help to apply simple relaxation techniques accompanied by respiratory patterns. Relaxing the body muscularly releases more endorphins that limit painful sensations.

Postures for Relaxation

Place yourself in a position that facilitates relaxation. You can use several cushions and pillows to do so.

There are several postures that help the body be more comfortable and without tension. The most suitable ones are: stretched in a lateral position, kneeling in a prone position, and sitting in a chair. Being in a supine position with your legs raised, flexed, and placed on a chair is also a suitable position, although it should be taken into account that from month six, supine postures may not be suitable.

In a **lateral position**, the abdomen is more relaxed and breathing is easier.

In this position, we stretch on the floor on our side with legs bent. Place a folded cushion or blanket underneath your head and another cushion or blanket between your knees.

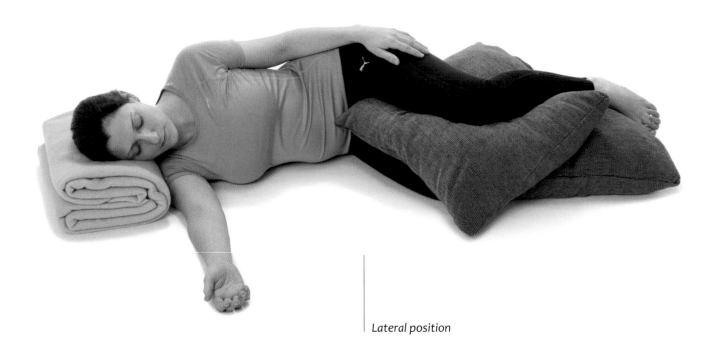

Lateral position

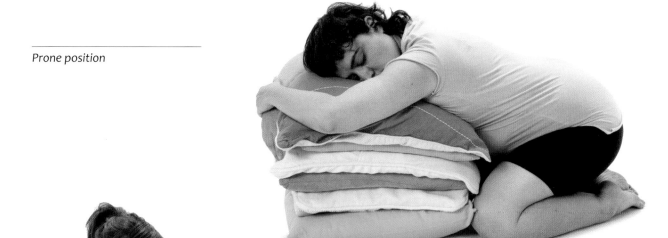

Prone position

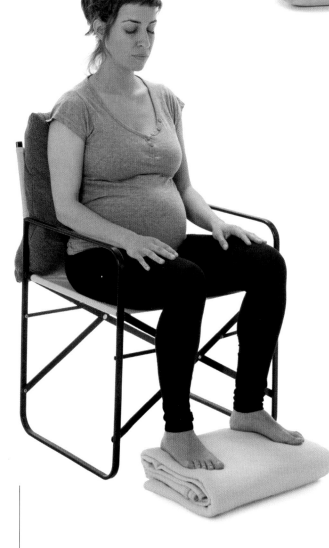

Sit on a chair.

Kneeling in a **prone position** relieves hip, groin, and lumbar tension and discomfort, allowing your back to relax.

In this position, place several pillows on the floor. Kneel with your legs apart and rest your chest, abdomen, and face on the pillows. Move your glutes toward your heels and surround the pillows with arms relaxed.

Sitting **on a chair** helps keep you more awake so you can practice visualization.

In this position, keep your back straight, resting on the back of the chair. A cushion can be placed behind the lumbar area to ensure your lumbar area is supported and resting. Keep your head straight and aligned with your body with your chin gently inward. Place your feet forward, parallel to each other and slightly spaced apart. If your feet do not reach the floor, it is advisable to place a pillow, firm cushion, or other support under your feet. Rest your hands on your thighs.

- Regulates metabolism, heart rate, and breathing.

- Frees you from tension, helps you sleep better.

- Reduces stress, relieves anxiety.

- Along with respiratory techniques, relaxation is a useful tool for pain and tension control in labor.

Relaxation Technique

To begin the relaxation, find a quiet place with a pleasant temperature.

Relaxation begins by closing your eyes. Observe the rhythmic movement of your abdomen as you breathe in and breathe out. Be conscious of the air coming in and out of your nostrils. With each exhalation, loosen your body more and more.

We become aware of the present moment, of the place in which you are in, and of your own body.

Go through the different parts of the body, without rushing, one by one, feeling them and helping them to relax little by little.

- ◆ Begin by paying attention to your right foot. Tense and then and release it, relaxing the toes, the sole, the heel, and the back. Do the same for your ankle, calf, knee, and right thigh.

- ◆ Repeat the process with your left foot and leg.

- ◆ Pay attention to your right hand. Separate your fingers slightly from each other. Release your hand and relax the palm and back of the hand. Continue to loosen your wrist, forearm, elbow, arm, and right shoulder.

- ◆ Repeat the process with your left hand and arm.

Relaxation is a beneficial practice for pregnant women and their babies. It soothes, calms, and improves the immune system and health.

- ◆ Shift your awareness to the base of your spine. Tense the muscles of your pelvic floor, relaxing your abdomen, hips, waist, and chest.

- ◆ Continue with your back, bringing your consciousness to your lower back and loosening it. Do the same with the dorsal and cervical parts.

- ◆ Finally, release the head and face: forehead, eyebrows, eyelids, nose, cheekbones, cheeks, and chin. Finish by separating the lips and tensing the jaw.

Now you can feel the whole body is fully relaxed. Stay quietly for a few minutes in silence, observing your slow and paused breathing.

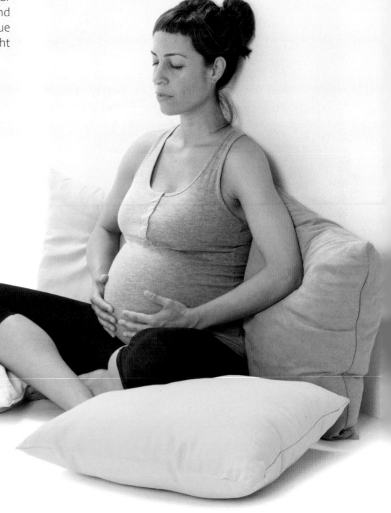

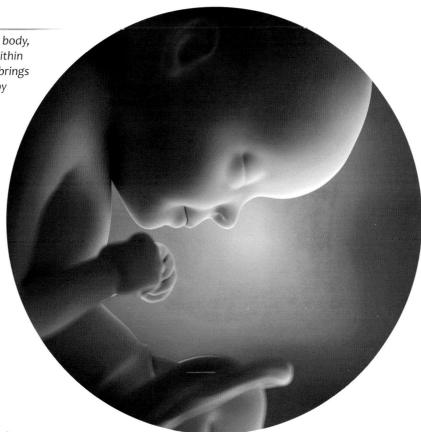

Visualizing the baby's body, developing placidly within the mother's uterus, brings confidence to the baby and the mother.

Visualization Technique

Visualization is a technique that uses one's own imagination to achieve goals, such as reducing stress and improving health. Imagination gives us the ability to create a mental image.

The ideal time to start a visualization is after relaxing. During visualization, the attention is directed toward the inside and, little by little, the mind can reach a state of great calm. The higher this state, the easier it is to create images.

Through imagination, we can visualize the baby inside the uterus to send them serenity and peace.

- Start by placing your hands on your abdomen to come into more direct contact with your baby. Visualize their silhouette submerged in the amniotic fluid, imagine the atmosphere that surrounds them, and feel how they are protected by water.

- Continue to visualize their face, closed eyes, nose, ears, and whole face. Now look at their little hands, feet, and body. Imagine how their whole body is forming in a harmonic way.

- We felt they are quiet and relaxed. Let's wrap them in a warm embrace full of love and gratitude.

- Spend a few minutes breathing slowly, with confidence in the process of life.

Leave this meditative state little by little. It is advisable to move your hands, feet, and head slowly, finally opening your eyes, while taking deeper and more complete breaths. Let out sighs and yawns. With this sense of well-being and renewed energies, we can return to our daily life.

Glossary

Braxton Hicks contractions. These are contractions that prepare the body for childbirth. They are not labor contractions. They are usually noticed in the third trimester in the form of tension in the belly. They are irregular and are not painful.

Kegel exercises. These consist of contracting the pelvic muscles up and in for a few seconds, repeating the process several times. This exercise strengthens the pelvic floor.

Afterpain. Contractions of the uterus due to oxytocin that is produced by stimulating the breasts during lactation.

Isometric stretching. In an isometric stretch, the muscle becomes tense but does not change in length. Isometric contraction of a muscle can occur at the most eccentric position, for example, at the longest length or stretch of the muscle.

Supine hypotension. When lying on your back, the weight of the uterus exerts pressure on the veins producing a feeling of dizziness. If you do not have any problems, supine stretches may be performed until the last six weeks of pregnancy.

Lochia. Fluids that present themselves in the form of short and scarce menstruation produced by uterus lining elimination after childbirth.

Oxytocin. This is a hormone that stimulates the smooth muscle of the uterus causing it to contract during childbirth. It is responsible for the secretion of breast milk.

Pubic symphysis. This is a joint that joins the two branches of the pelvis and that is usually altered in pregnant women. Its mobility can cause problems if exercises are performed that strain it (pubic diastasis).

Bibliography

BARBIRA-FREEDMAN, Françoise. *Yoga for pregnancy, childbirth and more. (Yoga para embarazo, parto y más.)* Blume, Madrid, 2005.

BERG, Kristian. *Illustrated guide to therapeutic stretching. (Guía ilustrada de los estiramientos terapéuticos.)* Tutor Editorial, Madrid, 2012.

BONAMUSA, Marc. *Objective Flat Belly. (Objetivo vientre plano.)* Amat Editorial, Barcelona, 2016.

BUCHHOLZ, Sabine. *Gymnastics for pregnant women. (Gimnasia para embarazadas.)* Paidotribo, Barcelona, 2002.

CALAIS-GERMAIN, Blandine. *Giving birth in motion. Pelvic mobilities in childbirth. (Parir en movimiento. Las movilidades de la pelvis en el parto.)* La liebre de marzo, Barcelona, 2015.

CALAIS-GERMAIN, Blandine. *Safe Abs. (Abdominales sin riesgo.)* La liebre de marzo, Barcelona, 2010.

Charlish, ANNE. *Your Natural Pregnancy. (Tu embarazo natural.)* Paidotribo, Barcelona, 1995.

COCA, Isabel. *Ioga i gestació.* Publications of the Montserrat Abbey, Barcelona, 2019.

DEANS, Anne. *The Pregnancy Bible (La Biblia del embarazo).* Grijalbo, Barcelona, 2004.

DE GASQUET, Bernadette. *Abs: Stop the massacre! (Abdominales: ¡detén la masacre!)* RBA Books, Barcelona, 2015.

FERNÁNDEZ ARRANZ-LAMBRUSCHINI-FERNÁNDEZ ARRANZ, Mayte, Roberto, Julita. *Pilates Handbook applied to pregnancy (Manual de Pilates aplicado al embarazo).* Panamericana, Madrid, 2016.

FERNÁNDEZ ARRANZ-LAMBUSCHINI-FERNÁNDEZ ARRANZ, Mayte, Roberto, Julita. *Postpartum Recovery. (Recuperación postparto).* Panamericana, Madrid, 2020.

FISCHER, Hanna. *Practical guide for labor preparation. (Manual práctico de preparación al parto.)* McGraw-Hill, Madrid, 2008.

GARCÍA MARTIN-LÓPEZ MAZARIAS, Esther, Bélen. *Your pelvic floor in shape (Tu suelo pélvico en forma).* Arcopress, 2019.

ISACOWITZ-CLIPPINGER, Rael, Karen. *Pilates Anatomy. (Anatomía del pilates).* Tutor Publications, Madrid, 2020.

IYENGAR-KELLER-KHATTAB, Geeta, Rita, Kerstin. *Iyengar Yoga for Motherhood.* Sterling Publishing, New York, 2010.

JEAN COSNER-MALIN, Holly, Stacy. *Pilates with your baby. (Pilates con tu bebé.)* Oniro Publications, Barcelona, 2006.

STAUGAARD-JONES, Jo Ann. *Exercise and Movement Anatomy. (Anatomía del ejercicio y el movimiento.)* Paidotribo, Barcelona, 2014.

KING-GREEN, Michael, Yolande. *The Pilates Method for Pregnancy (El método Pilates para el embarazo).* Paidos Ibérica, Barcelona, 2004.

MACKIN, Deborah. *Redefine your Figure. (Recupera tu figura).* Pearson, Madrid, 2003.

NELSON-KOKKONEN, Arnold, Jouko. *Stretching Anatomy. (Anatomía de los estiramientos.)* Tutor, Madrid, 2007.

RAMON GOMARIZ, Jorge. *Muscular Chain Stretches. (Estiramientos de cadenas musculares).* La liebre de marzo, Barcelona, 2009.

RIAL-PINSACH, Tamara, Piti. *Hypopressive Exercises (Ejercicios hipopresivos).* La Esfera de los Libros, Madrid, 2015.

ROBINSON-BRADSHAW-GARDNER, Lynne, Lisa, Nathan. *Pilates.* Blume, Barcelona, 2012.

SEIJAS, William. *Anatomy and Essential Stretches. (Anatomía y estiramientos esenciales).* Paidotribo, Barcelona, 2015.

SCATTERGOOD, E. *Gymnastics for Pregnant Women. (Gimnasia para embarazadas).* Hispano Europea, Barcelona, 2004.

STOPPARD, Miriam. *The new book of pregnancy and birth (El nuevo libro del embarazo y nacimiento).* Grijaldo, Barcelona, 2005.

WESSELS-OELLERICH, Miriam, Heike. *Gymnastics for pregnant women. (Gimnasia para embarazadas.)* Editorial Hispano Europea, Barcelona, 2005.